CURRENT TOPICS IN CHIKUNGUNYA

Edited by **Alfonso J. Rodriguez-Morales**

Current Topics in Chikungunya
http://dx.doi.org/10.5772/60827
Edited by Alfonso J. Rodriguez-Morales

Contributors

Dorothée Missé, Manuel Perera-Lecoin, Natthanej Luplertlop, Pornapat Surasombatpattana, Florian Liégeois, Rodolphe Hamel, Supatra Thongrungkiat, Ronald Enrique Morales Vargas, Hans Yssel, Shama Parveen, Farah Deeba, Nazia Afreen, Asimul Islam, Shobha Broor, Anwar Ahmed, Irshad Naqvi, Shivakumar Muthugounder S, Karthi S, Sarita Kumar, Dayron Fernando Martinez Pulgarin, Diego Zamora, Diana Muñoz, Cecilia Perret, Patrick Gérardin, Alfonso J. Rodriguez-Morales

Published by InTech

Janeza Trdine 9, 51000 Rijeka, Croatia

Publishing Process Manager Iva Simcic

Technical Editor SPi Global

Cover InTech Design team

First published September, 2016

Printed in Croatia

Additional hard copies can be obtained from orders@intechopen.com

Current Topics in Chikungunya, Edited by Alfonso J. Rodriguez-Morales

p. cm.

Print ISBN 978-953-51-2594-5

Online ISBN 978-953-51-2595-2

For EU product safety concerns:
IN TECH d.o.o., Prolaz Marije Krucifikse Kozulić 3, 51000 Rijeka, Croatia,
info@intechopen.com or visit our website at intechopen.com.

Meet the editor

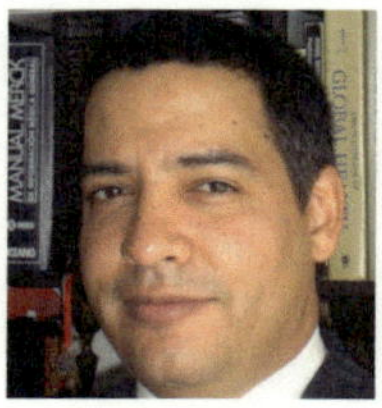

Dr. Alfonso J. Rodriguez-Morales is an expert in tropical diseases, particularly in Zoonotic and Vector-Borne Diseases. His research interests over the past years have been focused on malaria, Chagas disease, leishmaniasis, dengue, Zika and chikungunya, coordinating the Colombian Collaborative Network on Zika (RECOLZIKA). He is President of the Travel Medicine Committee of the Pan American Infectious Diseases Association (API), as well as Secretary of the Colombian Infectious Diseases Association (ACIN). Since 2014 he has been recognized as Senior Researcher by the national agency of Sicence in Colombia, Colciencias. He is Professor and Appointed Director of Research of the Faculty of Health Sciences of the Universidad Tecnológica de Pereira in Pereira, Risaralda, Colombia. His H index is currently 17.

Contents

Preface

Chikungunya has become an important cause of morbidity, although with a low mortality in certain areas of the world - the tropical (mainly due to vector-borne transmission) and non-tropical areas (due to sporadic vector-borne transmission and mother-to-child transmission) - occurring in rural and urban settings (1-3). Just in Colombia, during 2014–2015, more than 3 million cases were estimated to have occurred, including severe and atypical cases as well as deaths, including pregnant and newborn cases with congenital disease (4-6). In addition to acute disease and subacute and chronic manifestations, today known as post-chikungunya chronic inflammatory rheumatism (pCHIK-CIR) is an important condition which compromises half of the patients who have suffered this arboviral disease mainly in La Reunión, France, India, and Colombia (3, 7-9). For all these reasons, research on this arboviral disease is of utmost relevance particularly in endemic settings, mostly in developing countries, and particularly in Latin America. However, exposure to the virus in these areas in the context of globalization also gains importance given the increasing number of imported cases (10-13), even with the risk of autochthonous transmission as have occurred in the Mediterranean areas of Europe, such as in South France, Eastern Spain, or Northwestern Italy (14). As with other neglected arboviruses, chikungunya deserves more research and multiple new approaches for its study. More approaches with the vision of "One Health" are clearly necessary (15). Also, more interaction between medical doctors and doctors of veterinary medicine, as the role of animal reservoirs in chikungunya, is still, by far, unknown. Holistic control approach requires both of them involved, especially because most of the burden related to chikungunya and other neglected arboviral diseases (Mayaro, Usutu, Kyasanur, Oropouche, among others), would be avoidable (16). Now, there is the emergence of Zika, which can even lead to deaths, too (17-21).

With these conceptions in mind, this book includes different topics with regard to epidemiology, biology, clinical manifestations, treatment, and prevention, including entomological aspects of the wide spectrum of manifestations caused by the chikungunya virus infection, trying to update the most significant research in many of them as well as to offer a multinational perspective on different aspects. This book has been organized in two major sections: (I) "Clinical and Epidemiological Aspects" and (II) "Entomology." Section I includes topics covering epidemiological and clinical experience and studies in Colombia, Chile, Mexico, La Reunión, France, and India, including the infection during pregnancy and children, imported cases, ocular manifestations, coinfections, and therapeutics. Section II includes topics covering entomological aspects, related to vector control, and new options for biological control of *Aedes aegypti,* the main vector of chikungunya.

Commissioning of this book has been related in part to my recent involvement in chikungunya research, making the first publications of Colombia, as well as among the first in Latin

America about multiple aspects of this arboviral disease. Part of this is a clear reflection of the work impulse at the Research Group Infection Public Health and Infection of the Faculty of Health Sciences of Universidad Tecnológica de Pereira, directed by Dr. Guillermo Javier Lagos-Grisales, not just a partner and a colleague, but mainly a friend and an extreme believer in our work.

Following the same philosophy that we had on my three previous books with InTech, *Current Topics in Tropical Medicine* (22), *Current Topics in Public Health* (23), and *Current Topics in Echinococcosis* (24), this book does not intend to be an exhaustive compilation, and this first edition has included not just multiple different topics but also a wide geographical participation from many countries of different regions of the world. Its online availability through the website of InTech, as well as the possibility to upload the complete book or their chapters in personal websites and institution repositories, allows it to reach a wide audience.

I would like to give a very especial thanks to InTech (for the fourth time), and particularly to Iva Simcic (Publishing Process Manager), for the opportunity to edit this interesting and important book, as well as for their constant support.

I want to take the appropriate time and space, as I used to do, to dedicate this book to my beloved family (Aurora, Alfonso José, Alejandro, and Andrea, the neurologist) and particularly to my lovely wife, Diana. After 5 years together, I am so certain she is everything to me. She is the engine of my life. And due to her support, projects like this one would be not only just possible, but also successful. She is the highest blessing in my life, my soul mate, and my strongest support for any journey; she provides everything in my life, day to day. Also I would like to thank my friends and my undergraduate and postgraduate students of health sciences in Colombia, Venezuela, and around Latin America. It is time to say thanks to my colleagues at the Working Group on Zoonoses, the International Society for Chemotherapy, and the Committee on Zoonoses and Haemorrhagic Fevers of the Colombian Infectious Diseases Society (ACIN), and to more than 40 members of our Colombian Collaborative Network on Zika (RECOLZIKA) (www.RECOLZIKA.org), which I have the pleasure to chair, especially to my friends Wilmer E. Villamil-Gómez, Alberto Paniz-Mondolfi, and Jorge L. Alvarado-Socarras, among many others across Colombia and Latin America. I would like to thank Dr. Juliana Buitrago-Jaramillo, the former Dean of the Faculty of Health Sciences, Universidad Tecnológica de Pereira, who supported most of the efforts of our research group, Public Health and Infection. Special thanks to my friend and colleague Dr. Guillermo J. Lagos-Grisales, MD, MPH. Also I would like to thank the current Dean, Dr. Rodolfo Cabrales, who has been an enthusiast and supporter of our research activity. Members of our research group and incubator consist of young and enthusiastic medical students and some veterinary medical students, as well as young medical doctors, who are pursuing significant improvements in the understanding of the epidemiology of zoonotic, vector-borne, parasitic and, in general, infectious diseases, in our country with international projection. The year 2016 has been highly productive for this recognized group, which is positioning as a leader in infectious disease epidemiology research in the Coffee-Triangle Region and very soon in the country. One chapter was written by two of our graduates. Thanks to Dr. Mondragón, who helped in the critical review of the editor's chapter.

Finally, I hope our readers enjoy this publication as much as I did reading the chapters of *Current Topics in Chikungunya.*

References

[1] Alfaro-Toloza P, Clouet-Huerta DE, Rodriguez-Morales AJ; Chikungunya, the emerging migratory rheumatism. Lancet Infect Dis 2015;15(5):510-2. doi: 10.1016/S1473-3099(15)70160-X.

[2] Hidalgo-Zambrano DM, Jiménez-Canizales CE, Alzate-Piedrahita JA, et al.; Electrocardiographic changes in patients with chikungunya fever. Revista Panamericana de Infectología 2015;17(3).

[3] Rodriguez-Morales AJ, Cardona-Ospina JA, Villamil-Gomez W, et al.; How many patients with post-chikungunya chronic inflammatory rheumatism can we expect in the new endemic areas of Latin America? Rheumatol Int 2015;35(12):2091-4. doi: 10.1007/s00296-015-3302-5.

[4] Cardona-Ospina JA, Henao-SanMartin V, Paniz-Mondolfi AE, et al.; Mortality and fatality due to Chikungunya virus infection in Colombia. J Clin Virol 2015;70:14-5. doi: 10.1016/j.jcv.2015.07.001.

[5] Hoz JM, Bayona B, Viloria S, et al.; Fatal cases of Chikungunya virus infection in Colombia: Diagnostic and treatment challenges. J Clin Virol 2015;69:27-9. doi: 10.1016/j.jcv.2015.05.021.

[6] Villamil-Gomez W, Alba-Silvera L, Menco-Ramos A, et al.; Congenital Chikungunya Virus Infection in Sincelejo, Colombia: A Case Series. J Trop Pediatr 2015;61(5):386-92. doi: 10.1093/tropej/fmv051.

[7] Cardona-Ospina JA, Vera-Polania F, Rodriguez-Morales AJ; Chikungunya or not, differential diagnosis and the importance of laboratory confirmation for clinical and epidemiological research: comment on the article by Rosario et al. Clin Rheumatol 2016;35(3):829-30. doi: 10.1007/s10067-015-2995-x.

[8] Rodriguez-Morales AJ, Gil-Restrepo AF, Ramirez-Jaramillo V, et al.; Post-chikungunya chronic inflammatory rheumatism: results from a retrospective follow-up study of 283 adult and child cases in La Virginia, Risaralda, Colombia. F1000Res 2016;5:360. doi: 10.12688/f1000research.8235.2.

[9] Cardona-Ospina JA, Diaz-Quijano FA, Rodriguez-Morales AJ; Burden of chikungunya in Latin American countries: estimates of disability-adjusted life-years (DALY) lost in the 2014 epidemic. Int J Infect Dis 2015;38:60-1. doi: 10.1016/j.ijid.2015.07.015.

[10] Rodriguez-Morales AJ, Bedoya-Arias JE, Ramirez-Jaramillo V, et al.; Using geographic information system (GIS) to mapping and assess changes in transmission patterns of chikungunya fever in municipalities of the Coffee-Triangle region of Colombia during 2014-2015 outbreak: Implications for travel advice. Travel Med Infect Dis 2016;14(1):62-5. doi: 10.1016/j.tmaid.2015.06.009.

[11] Rodriguez-Morales AJ, Cardenas-Giraldo EV, Montoya-Arias CP, et al.; Mapping chikungunya fever in municipalities of one coastal department of Colombia (Sucre) using geographic information system (GIS) during 2014 outbreak: Implications for travel advice. Travel Med Infect Dis 2015;13(3):256-8. doi: 10.1016/j.tmaid.2015.05.007.

[12] Rodriguez-Morales AJ, Villamil-Gomez WE, Franco-Paredes C; The arboviral burden of disease caused by co-circulation and co-infection of dengue, chikungunya and Zika in the Americas. Travel Med Infect Dis 2016;14(3):177-9. doi: 10.1016/j.tmaid.2016.05.004.

[13] Jimenez-Canizales CE, Medina-Gaitan DA, Mondragon-Cardona AE, et al.; From imported to an endemic disease: impact of Chikungunya virus disease in the hospital epidemiology, Tolima, Colombia, 2014-2015. Recent Pat Antiinfect Drug Discov 2015;10(1):64-6.

[14] Noel H, Rizzo C; Spread of chikungunya from the Caribbean to mainland Central and South America: a greater risk of spillover in Europe? Euro Surveill 2014;19(28):20855.

[15] Rodriguez-Morales AJ, Schlagenhauf P; Zoonoses and travel medicine: "one world--one health". Travel Med Infect Dis 2014;12(6 Pt A):555-6. doi: 10.1016/j.tmaid.2014.11.003.

[16] Patino-Barbosa AM, Bedoya-Arias JE, Cardona-Ospina JA, et al.; Bibliometric assessment of the scientific production of literature regarding Mayaro. J Infect Public Health 2016;9(4):532-4. doi: 10.1016/j.jiph.2015.10.001.

[17] Martinez-Pulgarin DF, Acevedo-Mendoza WF, Cardona-Ospina JA, et al.; A bibliometric analysis of global Zika research. Travel Med Infect Dis 2016;14(1):55-7. doi: 10.1016/j.tmaid.2015.07.005.

[18] Rodriguez-Morales AJ; Dengue and chikungunya were not enough: Now also Zika arrived. Archivos de Medicina 2015;11(2). doi: 10.3823/1245.

[19] Arzuza-Ortega L, Polo A, Perez-Tatis G, et al.; Fatal Sickle Cell Disease and Zika Virus Infection in Girl from Colombia. Emerg Infect Dis 2016;22(5):925-7. doi: 10.3201/eid2205.151934.

[20] Rodriguez-Morales AJ; Zika: the new arbovirus threat for Latin America. J Infect Dev Ctries 2015;9(6):684-5. doi: 10.3855/jidc.7230.

[21] Sarmiento-Ospina A, Vasquez-Serna H, Jimenez-Canizales CE, et al.; Zika virus associated deaths in Colombia. Lancet Infect Dis 2016. doi: 10.1016/S1473-3099(16)30006-8.

[22] Rodriguez-Morales AJ. (Editor). Current Topics in Tropical Medicine. ISBN 978-953-51-0274-8. InTech, Croatia, March 2012.

[23] Rodriguez-Morales AJ. (Editor). Current Topics in Public Health. ISBN 978-953-51-1121-4. InTech, Croatia, May 2013.

[24] Rodriguez-Morales AJ. (Editor). Current Topics in Echinococcosis. ISBN 978-953-51-2159-6. InTech, Croatia, September 2015.

Prof. Alfonso J. Rodriguez-Morales
MD, MSc, DTM&H, FRSTMH(Lon), FFTM RCPS(Glasg), FACE, PhD(c)
Part-time faculty instructor, Risk Factors (Epidemiology) (Coordinator)
Department of Community Medicine, School of Medicine
Lecturer, Frontiers Research, School of Veterinary Medicine and Zootechnics
Faculty of Health Sciences, Universidad Tecnológica de Pereira, Pereira, Risaralda, Colombia
Lecturer, Postgraduate in Epidemiology, Fundación Universitaria del Área Andina
Seccional Pereira, Pereira, Risaralda, Colombia
Cochairman, Working Group on Zoonoses, International Society for Chemotherapy (ISC)
Secretary, Colombian Association of Infectious Diseases (ACIN)
Member of the Committee on Zoonoses and Hemorrhagic Fevers, ACIN
President, ACIN Chapter Coffee-Triangle Region
President, Committee on Travel Medicine
Pan American Association of Infectious Diseases
Senior Researcher, Colciencias (2015–2019)

Section 1

Clinical and Epidemiological Aspects

Chapter 1

Chikungunya, a Global Threat Currently Circulating in Latin America

Alfonso J. Rodriguez-Morales, Jaime Andrés Cardona-Ospina and Wilmer E. Villamil-Gómez

Additional information is available at the end of the chapter

http://dx.doi.org/10.5772/64808

Abstract

Chikungunya fever (CHIK) is a highly important arbovirosis currently established in Latin America and the Caribbean (LAC); its acute and chronic burden is an overlooked issue for policy makers. Disease spread control and proper management of chronic-derived sequelae do not seem like a realistic goal in short- and mid-term. The CHIKV circulating in the Western Hemisphere is closely related to strains from Philippines, China, and Yap (Federated States of Micronesia), and vertical and horizontal transmission of infection has been reported. Pathogenesis is still not well understood, and vaccines are under development yet. Here, we provide a summary of information regarding LAC spread of the disease from a public health, clinical and molecular perspective, particularly from the experience in Colombia.

Keywords: Chikungunya, Latin America, public health, molecular epidemiology, clinical manifestations

1. Introduction

Chikungunya fever (CHIK) is a highly important arbovirosis to Latin America and the Caribbean (LAC) because it is an infectious disease that have evolved from a simple threat to an established disease with acute and chronic burden to almost all the American continent, both mainland and overseas territories. Moreover, the presence of suitable ecological conditions in nontropical areas and our highly interconnected world have led to the report of cases in at least four continents in the world. CHIK is an arthritogenic fever that has arrived to stay in the Americas. After its introduction in 2013 to the island of Saint-Marteen (two autochthonous cases confirmed on December 6, 2013), it quickly spread through overseas Caribbean territories with autochthonous transmission (Martinique and Saint Marteen, December 19, 2013; Guadeloupe, December 24, 2013; Saint Berthelemy, December 31, 2013; and British Virgin Islands, January 15, 2014). Next, on February 21, the World Health Organization (WHO) confirmed the arriving of CHIK to mainland South America in French Guiana with seven confirmed cases (two autochthonous). Since then, the disease has spread over the entire continent. Until today, it continues accounting for important acute and chronic burden to the healthcare systems of the region [1–7]. For example, in Colombia, until June 2016, more than 16,000 new cases of CHIK have been reported.

Currently, almost every country in LAC has reported autochthonous transmission of CHIK, some of them in confined territories, but others such as Colombia, Venezuela, and Ecuador with a more generalized and intense disease transmission. Non-LAC territories have suffered the impact of travel and suitable ecological conditions with vector availability (*Aedes aegypti and Aedes albopictus).* The United States of America presently report mainland autochthonous disease transmission in Florida, and in Europe the vector is widely spread through Italy, the southern coast of Spain and France, and some areas of Switzerland, Croatia, Montenegro, Slovenia, Albania, Greece, and Romania [8]. Additionally, although previous CHIK cases have been reported in Europe, alongside the LAC outbreak, there were mainland reported cases in France and Spain in 2014 and 2015, respectively. On October 21, 2014, the National IHR Focal Point for France notified the WHO of four laboratory confirmed and locally acquired CHIK cases in Montpellier. The four cases occurred within a same family who did not have any history of traveling outside France or their district of residence, but who lived near to an imported case from Cameroon. This was the first time that locally acquired transmission of CHIK has been detected in France since 2010 [9]. On the other hand, on August 3, 2015, the WHO was notified by the National IHR Focal Point for Spain of a case of CHIK in the city of Gandia, Valencian Community. The patient, a 60-year-old man, had no history of travel outside the European Region. A regional laboratory identified him with the detection by ELISA of IgM titers and subsequent IgG seroconversion. However, the National Reference Laboratory failed to confirm these results and it apparently was a false positive [10]. Likewise on September 9, 2015, the Ministry of Health and Social Affairs of Senegal notified the WHO of the beginning of active circulation of chikungunya virus (CHIKV) on August 27 in the region of Kédougou, where the latest active circulation was reported between 2009 and 2010 [11].

As showed, CHIKV can easily be spread into areas where suitable ecological conditions are done. In 2016, 16,653 CHIK cases in LAC have been newly diagnosed, both suspected and confirmed (epidemiological week 7) [12]. By the same time, in 2014, there were 1980 cases, but the current data are only about 17% of the reported cases in the same epidemiological week in 2015. Although it is possible that CHIK cases this year would be importantly lower than the previous, attention must be paid because probably it is going to have an epidemiological behavior that resembles dengue with episodes of seasonal epidemic outbreaks. Moreover, after the arriving of Zika to the region, efforts must be oriented not only to vector control programs but to develop proper diagnosis, treatment, and follow-up strategies in order to grant management and assessment of acute and chronic symptoms. Chikungunya, dengue, and Zika are three arbovirosis that already pose an important burden to LAC healthcare systems. They have showed our weaknesses in managing infectious disease spread and taught us that viral emerging infectious diseases are more than febrile illnesses. The latent threat of introduction of other *Aedes* sp. transmitted arbovirosis, like Mayaro or other viral hemorrhagic fevers transmitted for arthropods, call our attention to learn lesson and to take planed actions.

2. Virology and molecular epidemiology

CHIKV is a member of the genus *Alphavirus,* family *Togaviridae,* that was first isolated from the serum of a febrile human in Tanganyika (Tanzania) in 1952–1953 [13,14]. However, reported cases from India and Japan have suggested that CHIKV epidemics could have occurred as early as 1779 [15]. Besides, after its isolation, the virus was found repeatedly in numerous countries in Central, Southern, and Western Africa, as well as in many areas of Asia, and it has caused multiple outbreaks and epidemics in Africa, Southeast Asia, and Southern Europe [16–18].

The CHIKV is an enveloped, spherical virus with a diameter of 60–70 nm. It has a RNA, positive sense, linear genome of 11.8 kb that resembles eukaryotic mRNAs; given that at the 5′ end, it has a methyl guanylate cap, which is a nonstructural poly-protein precursor, and at the 3′ end, it has a poly(A) tail [17]. The 5′ precursor is cleaved into nsP1, nsP2, nsP3, and nsP4, which are involved in the virus replication and have functions and structures that are shared by other alphaviruses [17,19–21]. The nsP1 protein functions as cytoplasmic RNA capping enzyme, the nsP2 protein is a cysteine protease with a partially constricted substrate-binding site and two separate domains with helicase and protease activity [20], the nsP3 protein is essential for negative strand RNA synthesis, and the nsP4 protein works as an RNA-dependent RNA polymerase [17–19,21]. The 3′ poly(A) tail consists of 26S mRNA whose products include the structural proteins: the surface glycoproteins (E1 and E2), the capsid protein, and small peptides (E3 and 6K). The surface glycoprotein E2 has a role in viral attachment, and the surface glycoprotein E1 is the fusion protein that facilitates the viral entry [18,19,22].

Currently, there are three CHIKV-identified genotypes based on the E1 gene and the full genome sequence: East/Central/South African (ECSA), West African, and Asian. Phylogenetic analyses suggest that CHIKV spread from Africa to Asia episodically [23,24] and that the CHIKV strains circulating in the Caribbean came from the >2005 Southeast Asian clade, which previously moved into Western and South Pacific (American Samoa and Yap) and then to the Western Hemisphere. The CHIKV circulating in the Western Hemisphere is closely related to strains from Philippines, China, and Yap (Federated States of Micronesia) [25–30]. By contrast, the circulation of the ECSA genotype has been confirmed in Brazil apparently imported from Angola [31]. During the current LAC epidemics, the virus has showed mutation rates that are in accordance with previous evolutionary rate model, which predicted approximately 10 nucleotide mutations over the entire genome during the course of a 1-year epidemic [23,26,30]. The LAC CHIKV possess two unique amino acid differences and a 12-nucleotide deletion that could be useful in future for tracking of this strain [26].

3. Pathogenesis and disease transmission

Conventionally, CHIKV transmission is considered to be through flying arthropods of the *A. aegypti* o *A. albopictus* species. However, evidence suggested that viable infective virus is excreted in the saliva of monkeys, mice, and humans, and it could be a source of infection particularly in immunocompromised patients [32,33]. Vertical transmission has also been reported [34,35]. Despite some studies failed to show effect of CHKV infection during pregnancy on major obstetrical outcomes or congenital anomalies, long-term follow-up studies have reported poor neurocognitive outcomes of newborns and even poorer results in patients with neonatal CHIKV encephalopathy [36,37].

After its entry to the human host, the CHIKV first replicates in the skin fibroblasts [38,39], next it enters to the circulatory system, and triggers an early type I interferon response [40]. Apparently, alterations in this response are associated with more severe disease and death [41]. Next, it disseminates from blood to various tissues, it lodges in immune-privileged niches, and it replicates in the joints and skeletal muscles that are associated with extensive inflammatory cell recruitment [38,40,42–45]. CHIKV infection can persist in mononuclear cells and macrophages that are another primary cellular target and help in virus dissemination and chronic articular symptoms [38,46,47]. It has been proposed that viral persistence is associated with expression of interferon (IFN)-α, interleukin (IL)-10, and monocyte chemotactic protein 1 (MCP-1 or CCL2) [40]. Chikungunya infection causes high levels of IFN-α, suggesting strong innate immunity, along with the production of IL-4, IL-10, and IFN-γ, suggesting the engagement of the adaptive immunity. Notably, circulating T lymphocytes showed a CD8+ T lymphocyte response in the early stages of the disease and a CD4+ T lymphocyte-mediated response in the later stages, and IFN-γ and IL-12 levels have been observed to rise dramatically during the acute phase of chikungunya fever. The level of IL-12 returns to normalcy in patients who recover. In contrast, patients who develop chronic arthritis show persistently high IL-12 levels. Histologic examination of synovia from patients with chronic arthritis following chikungunya fever has revealed joint inflammation due to macrophages containing viral material. Elevated expression of MCP-1, MCP-2, and MCP-3 has been associated with bone reabsorption and bone lose, and CHIKV seems to favor a pro-osteoclastic microenvironment disrupting the receptor activator of nuclear factor-κB ligand/osteoprotegerin (RANKL/OPG) ratio [43,48].

Support cells of the central nervous system, such as astrocytes and oligodendrocytes, have shown to be infected with CHIKV in human, primate, and mice models [49,50]. Apparently, the astrocytes play an important role in replicating the virus and are susceptible to die because of the infection, whereas the microglia seems to be infection-resistant [50]. The infected cells are induced to express high levels of cytokines and chemokines related to an upregulation on innate immune response [50,51]. The adaptive immune response apparently occurs early in the infection. Higher and early increase of IgG3 titers has been correlated with efficient viral clearance and long-term viral protection [52], whereas higher level of C-reactive protein is related to lymphopenia, lower monocyte level, neutrophilia, and high viral load [19,53].

4. Clinical manifestations and chronic sequelae

It was previously believed that asymptomatic seroconversion was a rare event. However, results point that the subclinical: symptomatic proportion is at least of 4.6:1 patients [54]. The clinical course of CHIK could be divided into three phases: acute, subacute, and chronic. The acute phase has usually been considered from the start of the symptoms (day 0) until the day 10. The most frequent symptoms are arthralgia, fever, and rash [28,55,56]. Other symptoms that could be present are headache, myalgia, pruritus, dizziness, nausea, vomiting, diarrhea, asthenia, red eyes, and although unusual, hemorrhagic symptoms could be present too [28]. The arthralgia usually is a bilateral and symmetric polyarthralgia of large joints that involves the appendicular skeleton; it is more severe in viremic patients, and the joints more frequently affected are of the lower limbs particularly, knees and ankles. Impairment of the finger joints is more frequent in women like the periarticular swelling too. Some patients can feel pain in previous bone fractures or ligament injuries as well as pain along ligament insertions and talalgia [57,58]. Likewise, skin involvement is important, although some studies reporting cutaneous manifestations are limited by the lack of confirmation of infection through serological test. Dermatological lesions comprise a wide spectrum. It could be morbilliform eruption, the most common type of lesion, scaling, confluent macular erythema, intertrigo, hypermelanosis, xerosis, excoriated papules, urticaria, petechial spots, and bullae, among others [58,59]. The macular erythematous rash could appear at fourth day of fever, while dengue rash appears between days 5 and 6, and in Zika fever it could appear on the first symptomatic day. Mucosal involvement has been reported, with aphthous ulcers in mouth, conjunctival injection, and nasal ulceration with nasal skin necrosis [60,61]. Similarly, CHIK cases could manifest with vasculitis in legs or nose with complications that could lead to amputation. Laboratory findings are often unremarkable; lymphopenia and thrombocytopenia could be present but are rare and slight elevation of hepatic aminotransferases could be observed [58]. During this time, there is a lot of overlap between symptoms caused by CHIK, dengue, and Zika, and for this reason differential diagnosis must be made through specific laboratory assessment (Specific IgM titers or RT-PCR) [62,63]. However, some features could help to guide clinical probability in field work. For instance, acute reactants such as C-reactive protein and sedimentation rate could be high, in contrast with dengue and Zika [64–103]. Cardiovascular assessment through electrocardiographic and echocardiographic imaging must be strongly considered. Ventricular and supraventricular arrhythmias and signs of myocarditis or acute effusive pericarditis could be present [104].

During the acute phase of the disease, some patients evolve to some clinical presentations that, because it is apparent rare occurrence, have been called "atypical manifestations" that include severe disease manifestations. These clinical manifestations include comprises in neurological, respiratory, cardiovascular, and cutaneous systems, among others that could evolve to death [3,61,64–68]. Older age and comorbidities are associated with the appearance of severe cases, death, and evolution to chronic forms of the disease [64]. Ocular manifestations are important too, being the anterior uveitis the most frequent, although retinitis and optic neuritis have also been reported [69]. During the outbreak of 2006 in Reunion Island, mortality attributable to CHIK was recorded, and during the LAC outbreak, fatalities have been noted with an estimated case fatality rate of 0.012% [3,64,65]. It is important to highlight that co-infection could be an issue where co-circulation of CHIK, dengue, and Zika has been reported since mixed clinical pictures could be present.

After 10 days of infection, the majority of patients will improve and symptoms will disappear, but there is a proportion of patients that will evolve to the subacute and chronic phase of the disease. The chronic phase is usually defined as the presence of symptoms at least for 2 or 3 months. The symptoms present during this phase affect quality of life and they can be derived from different involving systems [70]. According with previous estimates, 41.57% of CHIK-infected people would develop chronic inflammatory rheumatism (pCHIK-CIR), both arthritis and arthralgia, at 12 months [71]. Estimates derived from a systematic review and meta-analysis [105] showed, in the most conservative scenario, about 25% of CHIK would develop pCHIK-CIR, 34% considering the most representative studies, and 14% would develop chronic arthritis. Retrospective studies from cohorts in Colombia support these findings [72,73], but prospective studies are needed in order to establish the real risk of progression in LAC since geographical variation has been reported. When pCHIK-CIR appears, it usually involves ankles, knees, shoulder, and elbow [74]. And sometimes, it can mimic seronegative rheumatoid arthritis [75–77]. Although it is unknown if pCHIK-CIR is a lifetime condition, follow-up studies have found persistence of bone erosions and articular symptoms even after 6 years [78]. The risk of articular symptoms' persistence is apparently increased with older age, severity of initial joint pain, underlying osteoarthritis, gender (i.e. women), and number of comorbidities [64,70,79–81].

Although less well documented, there are other chronic worrisome sequelae that could be derived from CHIK. For example, chronic sequelae derived from post-CHIK Guillain-Barré or post-CHIK neuropsychiatric disorders such as anxiety or depression [66,67,82,83], vision defects from ocular involvement [69], or congestive heart failure from dilated cardiomyopathy associated with myocarditis [84]. Hence, although CHIK-burden is already worrisome, derived costs, both direct and indirect, are probably underestimations of the real problem. Healthcare systems of the affected areas must be aware of the possible chronic consequences of CHIK infection and efforts for prevention of infection must be done and proper follow-up of infected patients must be granted. The real scope of the problem is still unknown and more research is needed.

5. Treatment and antiviral development

Until today, CHIKV infection during the acute phase is treated with hydration, non–anti-inflammatory antipyretics (acetaminophen), and symptomatic relief through the use of antihistaminic drugs or lotions for pruritus control. When pain does not relief with usual analgesia, general measures such as alternating cycles of 10 minutes of cold and 20 minutes of warm each 8 hours could be used avoiding the prescription of corticoids or nonsteroidal anti-inflammatory drugs. Currently, there are no approved antivirals to treat the infection, but research in the field has been increasing. Some antiviral molecules, which act by blocking virus proteins important for virus replication, have been reported [85]. Polymerase inhibitors, mainly nucleotide, have been tested with difficulty because the core polymerase subunit nsP4, which is shared by other alphaviruses, is inactive on its own [21,85]. However, Faviparir (6-fluoro-3-hydroxy-2-pyrazinecarbox-amide), a nucleotide RNA-base analog inhibitor, is promising because it reduces CHIKV replication, as well as in other alphaviruses, in mice [86]. Likewise, efforts have been made in order to identify pharmacophore features of protease (nsP2) inhibitors [87]. Molecular modeling has been used in the identification of novel and selective inhibitors with one of them having encouraging features [88]. Other drugs, such as ribavirin, interferon, mycophenolic acid, or arbidol, with known antiviral activity against other pathogens have been proved in CHIKV infection and could potentially be used in treatment [85,89]. Equally, other drugs without conventional antiviral activity have been proposed for treatment. For instance, chloroquine has been suggested as a drug with prophylactic and therapeutic effects apparently by impairing endosomal-mediated virus entry during early stages of virus replication [90]. Other anti-parasite agents, such as ivermectin and a benzimidazole-derived drug, have showed effects on replication at early and late stages of infection [91,92]. Doxycycline combined with ribavirin effectively inhibited CHIKV replication and attenuated its infectivity in vivo in animal models [93]. Besides, some plant-derived products, such as green tea components, flavonoids, diterpene esters, and complex plant alkaloids, have showed antiviral activity against CHIKV [85,94–96].

For the chronic phase of the disease, particularly for articular symptoms, there is little high-quality evidence to guide treatment. Recommendations worldwide have suggested treating inflammatory articular symptoms in an early fashion as rheumatoid arthritis, and some disease-modifying antirheumatic drugs, such as hydroxychloroquine and methotrexate, have been proved in pCHIK-CIR appa rently with good results [77,97]. Glucosamine and chondroitin sulfate could be used to treat pain in patients with previous arthrosis, and those patients with neuropathic pain pregabalin could be prescribed. Treatment of other nonarticular pCHIK chronic sequelae have been poorly studied and reported, and there is no a clinical studied and approved drug for pCHIK-CIR risk reduction. Although studies suggest that passive immunization with monoclonal antibodies may help in CHIKV-infected patients who are at risk of severe disease or in neonates born from viremic mothers [85].

6. Vaccines, disease prevention and control

Although efforts have increased up to this moment, there is no an approved vaccine for CHIK prevention. There are several vaccine strategies proven in CHIK that comprises live attenuated virus, chimeric virus, DNA vaccines, viral vector vaccines, viral subunits, inactivated virus, and virus-like particles. All of them in preclinical phase trials are used in animal models, mainly mice [85,98]. As for other virus diseases, apparently the best choice for anti-CHIKV vaccination is a strategy using an attenuated live virus vaccine, and there are developed candidates. For instance, two mutant virus strains, with large deletions in either the nsP3 gene or in the entire 6K gene, proved to be genetically stable, attenuated, highly immunogenic, and able to confer durable immunity after a single immunization in mice [99]. Neutralizing antibodies recognize the epitopes in the E2 glycoprotein and therefore E2 is another vaccine candidate [100].

Besides, efforts have been made in order to improve vector control strategies. Implementation research has been conducted in LAC in order to find ways to improve use of prevention tools such as insecticide-treated nets and covers, education, social mobilization, and water storage cleaning [101,102]. The potential to prevent and control not only CHIK, but to dengue and Zika too, encourages to direct efforts in order to grant vector control. Likewise, recent studies have shown that vector co-infection with the bacterium *Wolbachia pipientis* impedes virus infection. This bacterium is maternally inherited and is a promising technology to control disease spread [103].

Author details

Alfonso J. Rodriguez-Morales[1,2,3,4,5*], Jaime Andrés Cardona-Ospina[1] and Wilmer E. Villamil-Gómez[2,5,6]

*Address all correspondence to: arodriguezm@utp.edu.co

1 Public Health and Infection Research Group, School of Medicine and School of Veterinary Medicine and Zootechnics, Faculty of Health Sciences, Universidad Tecnológica de Pereira, Pereira, Risaralda, Colombia

2 Committee on Zoonoses and Haemorrhagic Fevers, Asociación Colombiana de Infectología, Bogotá, DC, Colombia

3 Working Group on Zoonoses, International Society for Chemotherapy, Aberdeen, United Kingdom

4 Colombian Collaborative Network on Zika (RECOLZIKA), Pereira, Risaralda, Colombia

5 Infectious Diseases and Infection Control Research Group, Hospital Universitario de Sincelejo, Sincelejo, Sucre, Colombia

6 Programa del Doctorado de Medicina Tropical, Universidad de Cartagena, Cartagena, Universidad del Atlántico, Barranquilla, Colombia

References

[1] Pan American Health Organization. Chikungunya Situation in the Americas 2014 [cited 2016 22/02]. Available from: http://www.paho.org/hq/index.php?option=com_topics&view=readall&cid=5855&Itemid=40931&lang=en.

[2] Cardona-Ospina JA, Diaz-Quijano FA, Rodríguez-Morales AJ. Burden of chikungunya in Latin American countries: estimates of disability adjusted life years (DALY) lost in 2014 epidemic. Int J Infect Dis. 2015; 38:60-61.

[3] Cardona-Ospina JA, Henao-SanMartin V, Paniz-Mondolfi AE, Rodriguez-Morales AJ. Mortality and fatality due to chikungunya virus infection in Colombia. J Clin Virol. 2015;70:14-15.

[4] Cardona-Ospina JA, Rodriguez-Morales AJ, Villamil-Gómez W. Burden of chikungunya in one coastal department of Colombia (Sucre): estimates of disability adjusted life years (DALY) lost in 2014 epidemic. J Infect Public Health. 2015;8(6):644-646.

[5] Cardona-Ospina JA, Villamil-Gómez WE, Jimenez-Canizales CE, Castañeda-Hernándeza DM, Rodríguez-Morales AJ. Estimating the burden of disease and the economic cost attributable to chikungunya, Colombia, 2014. Trans R Soc Trop Med Hyg. 2015;109(12):793-802.

[6] Jimenez-Canizales CE, Medina-Gaitan DA, Mondragon-Cardona AE, Rodriguez-Morales AJ. Letter to editor: from imported to an endemic disease: impact of chikungunya virus disease in the hospital epidemiology, tolima, Colombia, 2014-2015. Recent Pat Antiinfect Drug Discov. 2015;10(1):64-66.

[7] Rodriguez-Morales AJ, Cardenas-Giraldo EV, Montoya-Arias CP, Guerrero-Matituy EA, Bedoya-Arias JE, Ramirez-Jaramillo V, et al. Mapping chikungunya fever in municipalities of one coastal department of Colombia (Sucre) using geographic information system (GIS) during 2014 outbreak: Implications for travel advice. Travel Med Infect Dis. 2015; 13(3):256-258.

[8] World Health Organization. Chikungunya in the WHO European Region Copenhagen: WHO; 2015 [cited 2016 22/02]. Available from: http://www.euro.who.int/__data/assets/pdf_file/0005/246164/Fact-sheet-Chikungunya-Eng.pdf?ua=1.

[9] World Health Organization. Chikungunya – France 2014 [cited 2016 22/02]. Available from: http://www.who.int/csr/don/23-october-2014-chikungunya/en/.

[10] World Health Organization. Chikungunya – Spain (update) 2015 [cited 2016 22/02]. Available from: http://www.who.int/csr/don/17-september-2015-chikungunya/en/.

[11] World Health Organization. Chikungunya – Senegal 2015 [cited 2016 22/02]. Available from: http://www.who.int/csr/don/14-september-2015-chikungunya/en/.

[12] Pan American Health Organization. Number of reported cases in the countries of Americas (2016) (by weeks). Pan American Health Organization; 2016. p. 1.

[13] Karabatsos N. International catalogue of arthropod-borne viruses. San Antonio (TX): American Society for Tropical Medicine and Hygiene. 1985;3.

[14] Mason PJ, Haddow AJ. An epidemic of virus disease in Southern Province, Tanganyika Territory, in 1952-53; an additional note on chikungunya virus isolations and serum antibodies. Trans R Soc Trop Med Hyg. 1957;51(3):238-240.

[15] Carey DE. Chikungunya and dengue: a case of mistaken identity? J Hist Med Allied Sci. 1971;26(3):243-262.

[16] Powers AM, Brault AC, Tesh RB, Weaver SC. Re-emergence of chikungunya and O'nyong-nyong viruses: evidence for distinct geographical lineages and distant evolutionary relationships. J Gen Virol. 2000;81(Pt 2):471-479.

[17] Solignat M, Gay B, Higgs S, Briant L, Devaux C. Replication cycle of chikungunya: a re-emerging arbovirus. Virology. 2009;393(2):183-197.

[18] Powers AM, Logue CH. Changing patterns of chikungunya virus: re-emergence of a zoonotic arbovirus. J Gen Virol. 2007;88(Pt 9):2363-2377.

[19] Deeba F, Islam A, Kazim SN, Naqvi IH, Broor S, Ahmed A, et al. Chikungunya virus: recent advances in epidemiology, host pathogen interaction and vaccine strategies. Pathog Dis. 2016;74(3).

[20] Golubtsov A, Kaariainen L, Caldentey J. Characterization of the cysteine protease domain of Semliki Forest virus replicase protein nsP2 by in vitro mutagenesis. FEBS Lett. 2006;580(5):1502-1508.

[21] Rubach JK, Wasik BR, Rupp JC, Kuhn RJ, Hardy RW, Smith JL. Characterization of purified Sindbis virus nsP4 RNA-dependent RNA polymerase activity in vitro. Virology. 2009;384(1):201-208.

[22] Abere B, Wikan N, Ubol S, Auewarakul P, Paemanee A, Kittisenachai S, et al. Proteomic analysis of chikungunya virus infected microgial cells. PLoS One. 2012;7(4):e34800.

[23] Volk SM, Chen R, Tsetsarkin KA, Adams AP, Garcia TI, Sall AA, et al. Genome-scale phylogenetic analyses of chikungunya virus reveal independent emergences of recent epidemics and various evolutionary rates. J Virol. 2010;84(13):6497-6504.

[24] Santhosh SR, Dash PK, Parida MM, Khan M, Tiwari M, Lakshmana Rao PV. Comparative full genome analysis revealed E1: A226V shift in 2007 Indian chikungunya virus isolates. Virus Res. 2008;135(1):36-41.

[25] Lanciotti RS, Valadere AM. Transcontinental movement of Asian genotype chikungunya virus. Emerg Infect Dis. 2014;20(8):1400-1402.

[26] Lanciotti RS, Lambert AJ. Phylogenetic analysis of chikungunya virus strains circulating in the Western Hemisphere. Am J Trop Med Hyg. 2016.

[27] Gay N, Rousset D, Huc P, Matheus S, Ledrans M, Rosine J, et al. Seroprevalence of Asian lineage chikungunya virus infection on Saint Martin Island, 7 Months After the 2013 Emergence. Am J Trop Med Hyg. 2016;94(2):393-396.

[28] Mattar S, Miranda J, Pinzon H, Tique V, Bolanos A, Aponte J, et al. Outbreak of chikungunya virus in the north Caribbean area of Colombia: clinical presentation and phylogenetic analysis. J Infect Dev Ctries. 2015;9(10):1126-1132.

[29] Wang C, Saborio S, Gresh L, Eswarappa M, Wu D, Fire A, et al. Chikungunya virus sequences across the first epidemic in Nicaragua, 2014-2015. Am J Trop Med Hyg. 2016;94(2):400-403.

[30] Stapleford KA, Moratorio G, Henningsson R, Chen R, Matheus S, Enfissi A, et al. Whole-genome sequencing analysis from the chikungunya virus Caribbean outbreak reveals novel evolutionary genomic elements. PLoS Negl Trop Dis. 2016;10(1):e0004402.

[31] Teixeira MG, Andrade AM, Costa Mda C, Castro JN, Oliveira FL, Goes CS, et al. East/Central/South African genotype chikungunya virus, Brazil, 2014. Emerg Infect Dis. 2015;21(5):906-907.

[32] Gardner J, Rudd PA, Prow NA, Belarbi E, Roques P, Larcher T, et al. Infectious chikungunya virus in the saliva of mice, monkeys and humans. PLoS One. 2015;10(10):e0139481.

[33] Rolph MS, Zaid A, Mahalingam S. Salivary transmission of the chikungunya arbovirus. Trends Microbiol. 2016;24(2):86-87.

[34] Vasani R, Kanhere S, Chaudhari K, Phadke V, Mukherjee P, Gupta S, et al. Congenital chikungunya-A cause of neonatal hyperpigmentation. Pediatr Dermatol. 2015.

[35] Villamil-Gomez W, Alba-Silvera L, Menco-Ramos A, Gonzalez-Vergara A, Molinares-Palacios T, Barrios-Corrales M, et al. Congenital chikungunya virus infection in Sincelejo, Colombia: a case series. J Trop Pediatr. 2015;61(5):386-392.

[36] Fritel X, Rollot O, Gerardin P, Gauzere BA, Bideault J, Lagarde L, et al. Chikungunya virus infection during pregnancy, Reunion, France, 2006. Emerg Infect Dis. 2010;16(3):418-425.

[37] Gerardin P, Samperiz S, Ramful D, Boumahni B, Bintner M, Alessandri JL, et al. Neurocognitive outcome of children exposed to perinatal mother-to-child chikungunya virus infection: the CHIMERE cohort study on Reunion Island. PLoS Negl Trop Dis. 2014;8(7):e2996.

[38] Ekchariyawat P, Hamel R, Bernard E, Wichit S, Surasombatpattana P, Talignani L, et al. Inflammasome signaling pathways exert antiviral effect against chikungunya virus in human dermal fibroblasts. Infect Genet Evol. 2015;32:401-408.

[39] Schilte C, Buckwalter MR, Laird ME, Diamond MS, Schwartz O, Albert ML. Cutting edge: independent roles for IRF-3 and IRF-7 in hematopoietic and nonhematopoietic cells during host response to chikungunya infection. J Immunol. 2012;188(7):2967-2971.

[40] Hoarau JJ, Jaffar Bandjee MC, Krejbich Trotot P, Das T, Li-Pat-Yuen G, Dassa B, et al. Persistent chronic inflammation and infection by chikungunya arthritogenic alphavirus in spite of a robust host immune response. J Immunol. 2010;184(10):5914-5927.

[41] Couderc T, Chretien F, Schilte C, Disson O, Brigitte M, Guivel-Benhassine F, et al. A mouse model for chikungunya: young age and inefficient type-I interferon signaling are risk factors for severe disease. PLoS Pathog. 2008;4(2):e29.

[42] Ozden S, Huerre M, Riviere JP, Coffey LL, Afonso PV, Mouly V, et al. Human muscle satellite cells as targets of chikungunya virus infection. Plos One. 2007;2(6):e527.

[43] Herrero LJ, Taylor A, Wolf S, Mahalingam S. Arthropod-borne arthritides. Best Pract Res Clin Rheumatol.

[44] Labadie K, Larcher T, Joubert C, Mannioui A, Delache B, Brochard P, et al. Chikungunya disease in nonhuman primates involves long-term viral persistence in macrophages. J Clin Invest. 2010;120(3):894-906.

[45] Her Z, Malleret B, Chan M, Ong EK, Wong SC, Kwek DJ, et al. Active infection of human blood monocytes by chikungunya virus triggers an innate immune response. J Immunol. 2010;184(10):5903-5913.

[46] Gardner J, Anraku I, Le TT, Larcher T, Major L, Roques P, et al. Chikungunya virus arthritis in adult wild-type mice. J Virol. 2010;84(16):8021-8032.

[47] Poo YS, Nakaya H, Gardner J, Larcher T, Schroder WA, Le TT, et al. CCR2 deficiency promotes exacerbated chronic erosive neutrophil-dominated chikungunya virus arthritis. J Virol. 2014;88(12):6862-6872.

[48] Chen W, Foo SS, Taylor A, Lulla A, Merits A, Hueston L, et al. Bindarit, an inhibitor of monocyte chemotactic protein synthesis, protects against bone loss induced by chikungunya virus infection. J Virol. 2015;89(1):581-593.

[49] Abraham R, Mudaliar P, Padmanabhan A, Sreekumar E. Induction of cytopathogenicity in human glioblastoma cells by chikungunya virus. PLoS One. 2013;8(9):e75854.

[50] Das T, Hoarau JJ, Jaffar Bandjee MC, Maquart M, Gasque P. Multifaceted innate immune responses engaged by astrocytes, microglia and resident dendritic cells against chikungunya neuroinfection. J Gen Virol. 2015;96(Pt 2):294-310.

[51] Inglis FM, Lee KM, Chiu KB, Purcell OM, Didier PJ, Russell-Lodrigue K, et al. Neuropathogenesis of chikungunya infection: astrogliosis and innate immune activation. J Neurovirol. 2015.

[52] Kam YW, Simarmata D, Chow A, Her Z, Teng TS, Ong EK, et al. Early appearance of neutralizing immunoglobulin G3 antibodies is associated with chikungunya virus clearance and long-term clinical protection. J Infect Dis. 2012;205(7):1147-1154.

[53] Chow A, Her Z, Ong EK, Chen JM, Dimatatac F, Kwek DJ, et al. Persistent arthralgia induced by chikungunya virus infection is associated with interleukin-6 and granulocyte macrophage colony-stimulating factor. J Infect Dis. 2011;203(2):149-157.

[54] Yoon IK, Alera MT, Lago CB, Tac-An IA, Villa D, Fernandez S, et al. High rate of subclinical chikungunya virus infection and association of neutralizing antibody with

protection in a prospective cohort in the Philippines. PLoS Negl Trop Dis. 2015;9(5):e0003764.

[55] Dupuis-Maguiraga L, Noret M, Brun S, Le Grand R, Gras G, Roques P. Chikungunya disease: infection-associated markers from the acute to the chronic phase of arbovirus-induced arthralgia. PLoS Negl Trop Dis. 2012;6(3):e1446.

[56] Nkoghe D, Kassa RF, Caron M, Grard G, Mombo I, Bikie B, et al. Clinical forms of chikungunya in Gabon, 2010. PLoS Negl Trop Dis. 2012;6(2):e1517.

[57] Thiberville SD, Boisson V, Gaudart J, Simon F, Flahault A, de Lamballerie X. Chikungunya fever: a clinical and virological investigation of outpatients on Reunion Island, South-West Indian Ocean. PLoS Negl Trop Dis. 2013;7(1):e2004.

[58] Staikowsky F, Talarmin F, Grivard P, Souab A, Schuffenecker I, Le Roux K, et al. Prospective study of chikungunya virus acute infection in the Island of La Reunion during the 2005-2006 outbreak. PLoS One. 2009;4(10):e7603.

[59] Riyaz N, Riyaz A, Abdul Latheef EN, Anitha PM, Aravindan KP, Nair AS, et al. Cutaneous manifestations of chikungunya during a recent epidemic in Calicut, north Kerala, south India. Indian J Dermatol Venereol Leprol. 2010;76(6):671-676.

[60] Bandyopadhyay D, Ghosh SK. Mucocutaneous features of chikungunya fever: a study from an outbreak in West Bengal, India. Int J Dermatol. 2008;47(11):1148-1152.

[61] Torres JR, Cordova LG, Saravia V, Arvelaez J, Castro JS. Nasal skin necrosis: an unexpected new finding in severe chikungunya fever. Clin Infect Dis. 2015.

[62] Cardona-Ospina JA, Vera-Polania F, Rodriguez-Morales AJ. Chikungunya or not, differential diagnosis and the importance of laboratory confirmation for clinical and epidemiological research: comment on the article by Rosario et al. Clinical Rheumatology. 2016; 35(3): 829-830.

[63] Magurano F, Zammarchi L, Baggieri M, Fortuna C, Farese A, Benedetti E, et al. Chikungunya from the Caribbean: the importance of appropriate laboratory tests to confirm the diagnosis. Vector Borne Zoonotic Dis. 2015;15(4):258-260.

[64] Economopoulou A, Dominguez M, Helynck B, Sissoko D, Wichmann O, Quenel P, et al. Atypical chikungunya virus infections: clinical manifestations, mortality and risk factors for severe disease during the 2005-2006 outbreak on Reunion. Epidemiol Infect. 2009;137(4):534-541.

[65] de la Hoz JM, Bayona B, Viloria S, Accini JL, Juan-Vergara HS, Viasus D. Fatal cases of chikungunya virus infection in Colombia: diagnostic and treatment challenges. Journal of Clinical Virology. 2015;69(0):27-29.

[66] Lebrun G, Chadda K, Reboux AH, Martinet O, Gauzere BA. Guillain-Barre syndrome after chikungunya infection. Emerg Infect Dis. 2009;15(3):495-496.

[67] Villamil-Gomez W, Silvera LA, Paez-Castellanos J, Rodriguez-Morales AJ. Guillain-Barre syndrome after chikungunya infection: a case in Colombia. Enferm Infecc Microbiol Clin. 2016;34(2):140-141.

[68] Oehler E, Fournier E, Leparc-Goffart I, Larre P, Cubizolle S, Sookhareea C, et al. Increase in cases of Guillain-Barre syndrome during a chikungunya outbreak, French Polynesia, 2014 to 2015. Euro Surveill. 2015;20(48).

[69] Mahendradas P, Avadhani K, Shetty R. Chikungunya and the eye: a review. J Ophthalmic Inflamm Infect. 2013;3(1):35.

[70] Couturier E, Guillemin F, Mura M, Leon L, Virion JM, Letort MJ, et al. Impaired quality of life after chikungunya virus infection: a 2-year follow-up study. Rheumatology (Oxford). 2012;51(7):1315-1322.

[71] Rodriguez-Morales AJ, Cardona-Ospina JA, Villamil-Gómez W, Paniz-Mondolfi AE. How many patients with post-chikungunya chronic inflammatory rheumatism can we expect in the new endemic areas of Latin America? Rheumatol Int. 2015; 35(12): 2091-2094.

[72] Rodriguez-Morales AJ, Villamil-Gomez W, Merlano-Espinosa M, Simone-Kleber L. Post-chikungunya chronic arthralgia: a first retrospective follow-up study of 39 cases in Colombia. Clin Rheumatol. 2016; 35(3):831-832.

[73] Rodríguez-Morales AJ, Calvache-Benavides CE, Giraldo-Gómez J, Hurtado-Hurtado N, Yepes-Echeverri MC, García-Loaiza CJ, et al. Post-chikungunya chronic arthralgia: results from a retrospective follow-up study of 131 cases in Tolima, Colombia. Travel Med Infect Dis. 2016; 14(1):58-59.

[74] Chopra A, Anuradha V, Ghorpade R, Saluja M. Acute chikungunya and persistent musculoskeletal pain following the 2006 Indian epidemic: a 2-year prospective rural community study. Epidemiol Infect. 2012;140(5):842-850.

[75] Essackjee K, Goorah S, Ramchurn SK, Cheeneebash J, Walker-Bone K. Prevalence of and risk factors for chronic arthralgia and rheumatoid-like polyarthritis more than 2 years after infection with chikungunya virus. Postgrad Med J. 2013;89(1054):440-447.

[76] Foissac M, Javelle E, Ray S, Guerin B, Simon F. Post-chikungunya rheumatoid arthritis, Saint Martin. Emerg Infect Dis. 2015;21(3):530-532.

[77] Ganu MA, Ganu AS. Post-chikungunya chronic arthritis - Our experience with dmards over two year follow up. J Assoc Physicians India. 2011;59(2):83-86.

[78] Javelle E, Ribera A, Degasne I, Gauzere BA, Marimoutou C, Simon F. Specific management of post-chikungunya rheumatic disorders: a retrospective study of 159 cases in reunion island from 2006-2012. PLoS Negl Trop Dis. 2015;9(3):e0003603.

[79] Gerardin P, Fianu A, Michault A, Mussard C, Boussaid K, Rollot O, et al. Predictors of chikungunya rheumatism: a prognostic survey ancillary to the TELECHIK cohort study. Arthritis Res Ther. 2013;15(1):R9.

[80] Sebastian MR, Lodha R, Kabra SK. Chikungunya infection in children. Indian J Pediatr. 2009;76(2):185-189.

[81] Sissoko D, Malvy D, Ezzedine K, Renault P, Moscetti F, Ledrans M, et al. Post-epidemic chikungunya disease on Reunion Island: course of rheumatic manifestations and associated factors over a 15-month period. PLoS Negl Trop Dis. 2009;3(3):e389.

[82] Bhatia MS, Gautam P, Jhanjee A. Psychiatric morbidity in patients with chikungunya fever: first report from India. J Clin Diagn Res. 2015;9(10):Vc01-Vc03.

[83] Wielanek AC, Monredon JD, Amrani ME, Roger JC, Serveaux JP. Guillain-Barre syndrome complicating a chikungunya virus infection. Neurology. 2007;69(22): 2105-2107.

[84] Simon F, Paule P, Oliver M. Chikungunya virus-induced myopericarditis: toward an increase of dilated cardiomyopathy in countries with epidemics? Am J Trop Med Hyg. 2008;78(2):212-213.

[85] Ahola T, Courderc T, Ng LF, Hallengard D, Powers A, Lecuit M, et al. Therapeutics and vaccines against chikungunya virus. Vector Borne Zoonotic Dis. 2015;15(4): 250-257.

[86] Delang L, Segura Guerrero N, Tas A, Querat G, Pastorino B, Froeyen M, et al. Mutations in the chikungunya virus non-structural proteins cause resistance to favipiravir (T-705), a broad-spectrum antiviral. J Antimicrob Chemother. 2014;69(10):2770-2784.

[87] Singh Kh D, Kirubakaran P, Nagarajan S, Sakkiah S, Muthusamy K, Velmurgan D, et al. Homology modeling, molecular dynamics, e-pharmacophore mapping and docking study of chikungunya virus nsP2 protease. J Mol Model. 2012;18(1):39-51.

[88] Bassetto M, De Burghgraeve T, Delang L, Massarotti A, Coluccia A, Zonta N, et al. Computer-aided identification, design and synthesis of a novel series of compounds with selective antiviral activity against chikungunya virus. Antiviral Res. 2013;98(1):12-8.

[89] Di Mola A, Peduto A, La Gatta A, Delang L, Pastorino B, Neyts J, et al. Structure-activity relationship study of arbidol derivatives as inhibitors of chikungunya virus replication. Bioorg Med Chem. 2014;22(21):6014-6025.

[90] Khan M, Santhosh SR, Tiwari M, Lakshmana Rao PV, Parida M. Assessment of in vitro prophylactic and therapeutic efficacy of chloroquine against chikungunya virus in vero cells. J Med Virol. 2010;82(5):817-824.

[91] Mishra P, Kumar A, Mamidi P, Kumar S, Basantray I, Saswat T, et al. Inhibition of chikungunya virus replication by 1-[(2-methylbenzimidazol-1-yl) methyl]-2-oxo-indolin-3-ylidene] amino] thiourea(MBZM-N-IBT). Sci Rep. 2016;6:20122.

[92] Varghese FS, Kaukinen P, Gläsker S, Bespalov M, Hanski L, Wennerberg K, et al. Discovery of berberine, abamectin and ivermectin as antivirals against chikungunya and other alphaviruses. Antiviral Res. 2016;126:117-124.

[93] Rothan HA, Bahrani H, Mohamed Z, Teoh TC, Shankar EM, Rahman NA, et al. A combination of doxycycline and ribavirin alleviated chikungunya infection. PLoS One. 2015;10(5):e0126360.

[94] Lani R, Hassandarvish P, Chiam CW, Moghaddam E, Chu JJ, Rausalu K, et al. Antiviral activity of silymarin against chikungunya virus. Sci Rep. 2015;5:11421.

[95] Nothias-Scaglia LF, Pannecouque C, Renucci F, Delang L, Neyts J, Roussi F, et al. Antiviral activity of diterpene esters on chikungunya virus and HIV replication. J Nat Prod. 2015;78(6):1277-1283.

[96] Weber C, Sliva K, von Rhein C, Kummerer BM, Schnierle BS. The green tea catechin, epigallocatechin gallate inhibits chikungunya virus infection. Antiviral Res. 2015;113:1-3.

[97] Chopra A, Saluja M, Venugopalan A. Effectiveness of chloroquine and inflammatory cytokine response in patients with early persistent musculoskeletal pain and arthritis following chikungunya virus infection. Arthritis Rheumatol. 2014;66(2):319-326.

[98] Garcia A, Diego L, Judith B. New approaches to chikungunya virus vaccine development. Recent Pat Inflamm Allergy Drug Discov. 2015;9(1):31-37.

[99] Hallengard D, Kakoulidou M, Lulla A, Kummerer BM, Johansson DX, Mutso M, et al. Novel attenuated chikungunya vaccine candidates elicit protective immunity in C57BL/6 mice. J Virol. 2014;88(5):2858-2866.

[100] Brehin AC, Rubrecht L, Navarro-Sanchez ME, Marechal V, Frenkiel MP, Lapalud P, et al. Production and characterization of mouse monoclonal antibodies reactive to chikungunya envelope E2 glycoprotein. Virology. 2008;371(1):185-195.

[101] Caprara A, Lima JW, Peixoto AC, Motta CM, Nobre JM, Sommerfeld J, et al. Entomological impact and social participation in dengue control: a cluster randomized trial in Fortaleza, Brazil. Trans R Soc Trop Med Hyg. 2015;109(2):99-105.

[102] Quintero J, Garcia-Betancourt T, Cortes S, Garcia D, Alcala L, Gonzalez-Uribe C, et al. Effectiveness and feasibility of long-lasting insecticide-treated curtains and water container covers for dengue vector control in Colombia: a cluster randomised trial. Trans R Soc Trop Med Hyg. 2015;109(2):116-125.

[103] Johnson KN. The impact of Wolbachia on virus infection in mosquitoes. Viruses. 2015;7(11):5705-5717.

[104] Villamil-Gómez WE, Ramirez-Vallejo E, Cardona-Ospina JA, Silvera LA, Rodríguez-Morales AJ. Electrocardiographic alterations in patients with chikungunya fever from Sucre, Colombia: A 42-case series. Travel Med Infect Dis. 2016 (accepted, in press # TMAID-D-16-00072R1) doi: 10.1016/j.tmaid.2016.06.004

[105] Rodríguez-Morales AJ, Cardona-Ospina JA, Urbano-Garzón SF, Hurtado-Zapata JS. Prevalence of post-chikungunya chronic inflammatory rheumatism: a systematic review and meta-analysis. Arthritis Care Res (Hoboken) 2016. Epub Ahead March 25; available online at: http://onlinelibrary.wiley.com/doi/10.1002/acr.22900/abstract

Chapter 2

Chikungunya Fever During Pregnancy and in Children: An Overview on Clinical and Research Perspectives

Patrick Gérardin, A. Désirée LaBeaud, Nicole Ritz and Xavier Fritel

Additional information is available at the end of the chapter

http://dx.doi.org/10.5772/64424

Abstract

Chikungunya fever (CF) is an arboviral disease in worldwide expansion due to the plasticity of its pathogen and vector. Chikungunya virus (CHIKV), a positive-sense, single-stranded RNA alphavirus, is transmitted by *Aedes* (*Stegomyia*) *aegypti* and *Aedes albopictus* mosquitoes, two hegemonic anthropophilic day-biting mosquitoes capable of colonizing very different environments. This expert review discusses the molecular epidemiology, pathophysiology, clinical features, diagnosis, management, and prevention of CF during pregnancy, infancy, and childhood. Specifically, it will focus not only on the issue and challenges of perinatal mother-to-child transmission of CHIKV, its pathogenesis, and effects on neurodevelopment, but also on CHIKV-associated central nervous system disease in children, two previously ill-characterized features of the infection.

Keywords: Chikungunya virus, children, encephalitis, epidemiology, pregnancy

1. Introduction

Chikungunya fever (CF) is an arthropod-borne viral disease caused by the chikungunya virus (CHIKV) [1]. First described during an outbreak of dengue-like illness in the Newala district of the southern province of Tanganiyika (current Tanzania) in 1952–1953, the virus derives its name from the Makonde language and means "to become contorted" or "that which bends up" [2, 3]. These descriptors refer to the hallmark of the disease observed in adults, namely, severe incapacitating arthralgia, which was characterized as "frightening" in the seminal description of Robinson [4], as they lead to an inability to stand or walk [5]. In the majority of adult patients with CF, painful arthritis can continue for months and even years, yielding a significant persistent disease burden in affected populations [6–9]. CF is usually not life-threatening, although atypical and severe forms can occur during large-scale epidemics and a slight increase of mortality has accompanied the peak of the outbreak in La Réunion island [10–15]. Indeed, CHIKV-associated mortality is considered rare (~1‰ infections), but occurs primarily among the elderly, as evidenced in La Réunion, India, or in Puerto Rico [15–17].

Genome-scale phylogenetic analyses of CHIKV suggest that the virus originated from Africa and was subsequently introduced from Africa into Asia [18]. Phylogenetically, CHIKV has evolved into three distinct clades across the past five centuries: Asian, East Central South African (ECSA), and West African lineages.

In its natural cycle, CHIKV is transmitted by the bite of female arboreal *Aedes* (*Stegomyia*) mosquitoes. The peridomestic *Ae. aegypti*, the well-known vector of yellow fever and dengue, was identified as the primary vector of CHIKV during its inaugural outbreaks, both in Africa [2] and Asia [19]. It is only during the last decade that *Ae. albopticus* (also known as the Asian tiger mosquito) has been recognized as a new propagating vector of CHIKV [20]. Originally native to Southeast Asia, *Ae. albopticus* has adapted successfully to cooler climates and spread worldwide [21]. Alongside the broadening geographic distribution of this new hegemonic vector, genetic adaptation through mutations in the envelope glycoproteins E1 and E2 has led to increased infectivity and dissemination of CHIKV in *Ae. albopictus* [22]. Moreover, rapidly increasing international travel exposures has contributed to the global expansion of CF. Over the last decade, ECSA CHIKV has been responsible for most of the recorded cases worldwide; however, in late 2013 somewhat surprisingly Asian CHIKV emerged in the Caribbean island of Saint-Martin [23] and further spread to the neighboring islands and to the Americas, causing over 1.6 million cases by November 13, 2015 [24].

In addition to horizontal mosquito-borne transmission, CHIKV can also be transmitted vertically, and mother-to-child transmission of CHIKV infection often leads to severe neonatal disease, mostly encephalitis, that may cause lifelong disabilities [25]. This expert review will discuss the molecular epidemiology, pathophysiology, clinical features, diagnosis, management, and prevention of CF in the pregnant woman and in children, with a particular focus on the issue and challenges of congenital infection.

2. Molecular epidemiology

2.1. The chikungunya virus

CHIKV is a positive-sense, single-stranded RNA virus (genus Alphavirus, family Togaviridae), whose genome encodes at the 5′ extremity four nonstructural proteins (nsP_1, nsP_2, nsP_3, and nsP_4 responsible for negative-strand RNA synthesis, helicase and protease activity, RNA-dependent RNA polymerase activity, respectively) and at the 3′ extremity three envelope glycoproteins (E1, responsible for membrane fusion; E2, responsible for receptor binding and virulence (E1 and E2 carrying the main epitopes); E3, which serves as a clade-specific signal sequence for translocation of the glycoprotein complex in the endoplasmic reticulum) [26]. The native monomeric capsid is of ~40 nm diameter and the mature enveloped virion of ~70 nm, with a genome weighing ~11.8 kB. In recent years, the ECSA clade has selected the A226V substitution for better fitness to *Ae. albopictus* [27].

2.2. Chikungunya virus life cycle and modes of transmission

CHIKV is endemic in Africa where it circulates in sylvatic/enzootic cycle between arboreal mosquitoes (*Ae. furcifer, Ae. taylori, Ae. africanus,* and *Ae. luteocephalus*) and nonhuman primates and bats as reservoir hosts. Birds and other mammals have been found infected, but serve as occasional hosts without amplification of the virus [28]. In this context, the transmission depends on few mosquitoes and is usually clustered to sporadic cases [29].

In epidemic settings, the virus is transmitted by *Ae. albopictus* or *Ae. aegypti,* two day-biting anthropophilic vectors whose peak activity occurs early in the morning or in the evening, around or within human dwellings [20]. During the blood meal, *Aedes* mosquitoes acquire the virus from an infected person. In the subsequent extrinsic phase, the virus multiplies in the gut and migrates to the salivary glands (≥2 days depending on temperature) [30]. Further blood meals then transmit the virus to other individuals bitten (~4–5 feeds are needed to complete a successful blood meal for oviposition). *Aedes* spp. mosquitoes remain infectious throughout their whole life (30–45 days). Transmission between nonimmune human hosts is often massive and both sustained by densities of host and vector populations, very high titer viremias in humans, as well as by lack of protective host behaviors [29].

3. Pathophysiology

The onset of CF coincides with viremia (median duration: 5 days; range: 2–12 days). The mechanisms underlying acute CHIKV infection are still imperfectly understood [1]. Based on several animal models and meta-analysis of human immune signatures, once introduced into the dermis, it is believed that CHIKV disseminates in blood circulation causing a Th1-cytokine storm [31, 32]. CHIKV replicates in the liver hosted by endothelial and Küpffer cells, before reaching joint fibroblasts, muscle satellite, and skin epithelial cells, causing arthralgia, myalgia, and rash. Indeed, elective targeted sites where symptoms focus are typically infected, especially joint capsules, skeletal muscles, myotendinous insertions, and epidermis [1].

The intensity of the acute infection correlates with the CHIKV viral load [1]. The ability of CHIKV to disseminate through the body to the target organs is inversely correlated to the height of the host type-1 interferon (IFN) response. There is evidence that this CHIKV-specific innate immune response depends on the age and the maturity of the human host [33]. This can be shown in vulnerable persons by the breaking of two natural protective barriers, the blood brain barrier (BBB) and the skin barrier. Thus, infants and individuals >65 years of age are likely to exhibit severe or atypical localizations, including CHIKV-associated central nervous system (CNS) disease and severe bullous skin lesions. For example, the incidence of CHIKV-associated encephalitis is best described by an asymmetric U-shaped parabolic curve with the highest incidence occurring in infants below 6 months of age, the nadir being reached in young children (1–4 years of age), and a rise in seniors (≥65 years of age) to a figure five-fold lower than in infants [34]. Furthermore, skin blistering (rupture of bullous lesions) is almost exclusively observed in infants below 6 months of age [35].

B cells and neutralizing antibodies (abs) are critical for CHIKV clearance. Targeted epitopes for anti-CHIKV abs are located at C terminus of the E2 glycoprotein [36]. The contribution of lymphoid (CD_4 and CD_8) and other cell types responsible for the adaptive immunity could be critical in residual arthralgia. Their immaturity may explain the rarity of chronic arthralgia before the age of 3 years. The role of myeloid cells is less clear in the acute and chronic stage of human CHIKV infection. At the acute stage, blood monocytes may be able to disseminate the virus toward the target tissues [37]. At the chronic stage, myeloid cells may be involved in the clearance of infected cell debris but whether CHIKV replication, lack of virus antigen clearance, or both contribute to rheumatism deserves further studies.

The long-term persistence of CHIKV in tissue macrophages (aka "host sanctuaries") as main driver for chronic inflammation has been postulated from a single clinical observation [38]. It is supported by the data from several animal models (i.e., "for example, see [31]").

4. Clinical features

4.1. Chikungunya fever during pregnancy

Pregnancy, a situation physiologically oriented toward a Th2-lymhocyte shift [39], has not been associated as a condition precipitating severe forms of infection in CF [40].

The consequences for the mother and the fetus of a CHIKV infection acquired during pregnancy have been investigated extensively on La Réunion island, both in the Groupe Hospitalier Sud-Reunion cohort study [41, 42], in the CHIMERE ("Chikungunya Mère-Enfant") cohort study [43], and in the 2004–2006 Family Allowance Office (41,665 deliveries) and Mother and Child Welfare (42,259 neonates) records [44]. To date, there is no reliable epidemiological data linking CHIKV exposure in the first trimester of gestation to an increased risk for miscarriage, nor to any type of congenital malformation [43, 44].

In the second trimester, CHIKV infection has been associated with only three cases of antepartum fetal deaths without clear evidence for the mechanism [45]. The CHIKV crossing of the placenta may be accidental and the timing of the infections (12 weeks + 4 days, 15 weeks, and 15 weeks + 5 days) coincides in the woman with the period of deep trophoblast invasion. We hypothesize Toll-like receptor (TLR) 3 expression and Th1 cytokines associated with CHIKV infection could have disturbed the spiral arteries remodeling, characteristic of this particular period. Our hypothesis is supported by the involvement of TLR3 in both the susceptibility to CHIKV infection and the impairment of vascular remodeling or fetal losses, as demonstrated in mouse models [46, 47].

In the third trimester, although 14 cases of stillborn fetuses have been reported associated with CF in pregnant women cohorts [42, 43], none was positive for CHIKV, which supports the nonpermissiveness of the human syncytiotrophoblast to CHIKV, as suggested by data from the IFN-$\alpha/\beta R^{-/-}$ mouse model and the absence of infection of BeWo cell line [33]. These findings are strengthened by the data retrieved from French population-based records [44]. The contribution of subclinical premature placental abruption has been proposed to support the exceptional cases of prepartum CHIKV infection in preterm neonates [48].

Importantly, CHIKV can be transmitted vertically with a probability ~50%, when the parturient woman has a high viral load during the early stage of labor [41–43]. Fetal heart rate

http://dx.doi.org/10.5772/64424

decelerations and meconium-stained amniotic fluid are common during labor [42, 49]. Neither postponing delivery nor cesarean has been shown to be protective. In this context, the alleged mechanism to explain the transmission to the neonate is the breakdown of the syncytiotrophoblast due to uterine contractions (aka the "placental breeches" hypothesis) [42] while placental microtransfusion has not been ruled out by a proper scientific investigation.

There is no increased risk to the pregnant mother for hypertensive disorders, gestational diabetes mellitus, or intrauterine growth restriction associated with maternal CF [43, 44, 50]. The relationships between average fetal birthweight, small-for-gestational age, and the timing of maternal CF during pregnancy are displayed in Figure 1.

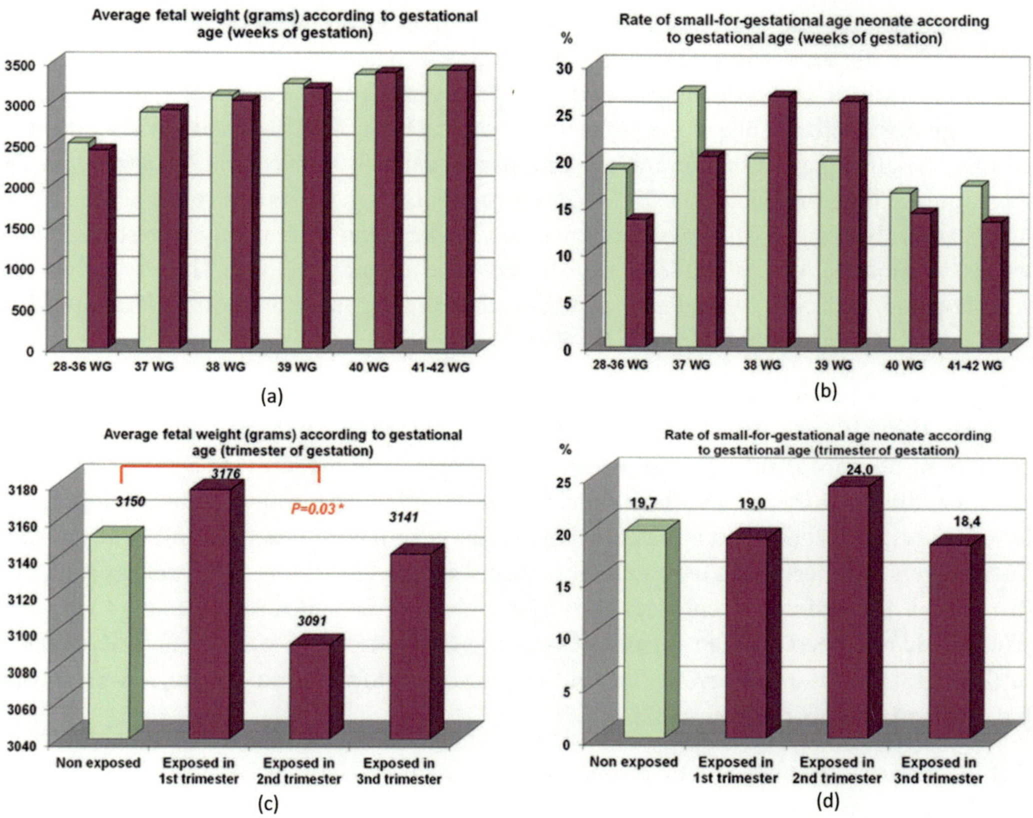

Liveborn neonates were matched on birth gestational age and further compared according to the timing of maternal chikungunya fever during pregnancy. There was no statistical difference between exposed (purple) and unexposed (green) neonates in terms of small-for-gestational age incidence and the only observed difference was a non-clinically relevant lower mean birthweight in neonates exposed in the second trimester of pregnancy (*).

Figure 1. Average fetal birthweight, small-for-gestational age and the timing of maternal CF during pregnancy, Reunion island 2006 (i.e., "for details see [50].").

Contrary to dengue [51, 52], there is also no increased risk for obstetric hemorrhage (placental abruption), preterm birth or low birthweight [43, 44, 50].

4.2. Chikungunya fever in the neonate ("congenital chikungunya")

Perinatal mother-to-child CHIKV infection was first reported during La Réunion island outbreak in year 2005 [53]. It has been investigated extensively on the island using both a retrospective regional case series [54] and two prospective hospital-based cohort studies, one on a local basis, the GHSR child cohort study [42], and the other on a regional basis, the "CHIMERE child" cohort study [55, 56].

Children who are prenatally infected with CHIKV are born with very low or even undetectable viremia, which makes the hypothesis of placental microtransfusion unlikely as the expected neonatal viremia would parallel the one of the mother. On average, it takes 4–5 days (range: 3–7 days) for the viral load of CHIKV transmitted at birth to reach a level significant enough to cause clinical disease. Neonatal CHIKV infection almost invariably presents with fever, pain, and suckling difficulties often requiring enteral or parenteral nutrition [42]. Other common symptoms include limb edema, *petechiae*, and a skin rash such as maculopapular rash and intertriginous aphthous-like ulcers [25]. Further clinical features of neonatal CHIKV infection, although relatively infrequent in this age group, are cyanosis (slate coloration) and hyperpigmentation of the skin [35, 50, 55, 57–61]. Their topography includes centro-facial area (nose, lips), trunk, abdomen, extremities, and knuckles. Hyperpigmentation may persist for several weeks to months. Vesiculobullous skin lesions are exceptional [62]. Thrombocytopenia, lymphopenia, and mild to moderate increases of serum aspartate aminotransferase (AST or SGOT) are frequent observations [42, 54, 57–61].

Life-threatening complications occur in half of the neonates and display two main clinical pictures: CHIKV-associated CNS disease (formerly reported as encephalopathy) that in fact consists of an encephalitis [34] and a multiple organ dysfunction (MOD) syndrome that combines a circulatory collapse (hypovolemia and hyperkinetic profile on echocardiography), lethargy, hemorrhages (disseminated intravascular coagulation), uremia, and cytolysis [59]. These severe manifestations require intensive care support including mechanical ventilation (for airway protection or neurosedation) in a quarter of neonates, vasoactive amines, and platelet and red blood cell transfusions. Risk factors for severe disease are immaturity and low birthweight. Indicators for severity include a reduced core to skin temperature, low prothrombin rate, and low platelet count [42].

The most characteristic magnetic resonance imaging (MRI) findings of the early acute stage (day 7), subacute stage (day 30), and chronic stage (day 120) of CHIKV-associated encephalitis are presented in Figure 2.

Changes in the course of cerebral edema and the passage from the cytotoxic to the vasogenic phase occur around day 10 of onset of neurologic symptoms and may be monitored by transfontanellar ultrasonography using velocimetry for measuring the blood flow in the anterior cerebral artery trunks (pericallosal and calloso-marginal arteries). Other neuroradiologic features include scattered supratentorial parenchymal lesions such as basal ganglia and subcortical area bleeding, but also the possibility of cerebellar hematoma, as a reversible consequence of DIC syndrome [42, 55, 60].

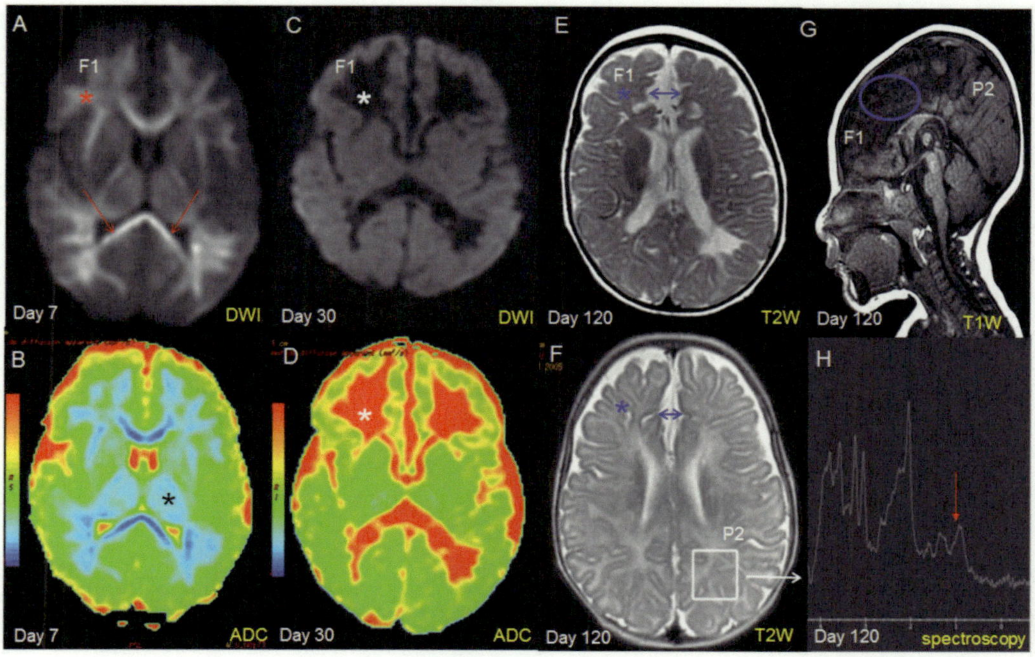

At day 7 of life, diffusion-weighted imaging (DWI) reveals scattered hyper-intensity signals of the white matter (WM), as marked in the frontal lobe (red star) or in the posterior arm of the corpus callosum (red arrows) evocative of cytotoxic edema (A), apparent diffusion coefficient (ADC) reveals low-output areas (blue) of restriction evocative of parenchymal ischemia (B). At day 30, DWI reveals scattered hypo-intensity signals of the WM in the same areas evocative of vasogenic edema (C), ADC reveals high-output areas of reperfusion (red) evocative of blood brain barrier leakage (D). At day 120, T2-weighted (T2W) and T1-weighted imaging (T1-W1) reveal a scattered scalloped appearance of the WM (blue star), a dilatation of the interhemispheric sulcus (double blue arrow) indicative of WM mass reduction (E,F), focused in the frontal (blue oval) lobe (G), monovoxel spectroscopy reveals a lower N-acetyl aspartate peak signal (red arrow) in the left posterior parietal lobe (P2) evocative of axonal loss (H).

Figure 2. Typical course of cerebral edema over a 4-month period in a neonate with CHIKV-associated CNS disease previously defined as "severe encephalopathy" [42], reclassified as CHIKV-associated encephalitis [34], Reunion island, 2006.

Transient coronary arteries dilatation was reported for six neonates [55]. Cardiologic involvement in this context is evocative of myocardiopathy or myocarditis, it includes left ventricular hypertrophy (sometimes complicated by left ventricular dysfunction or septal dyskinesia) and pericardial effusion [55, 61].

To date, only few CHIKV-associated deaths in neonates have been reported [55, 61, 62]. For the neonates without neurological involvement, recovery was observed in 1–3 weeks without *sequelae*; however, future long-term studies will shed more light on the presence of subtle morbidities related to CF in these infants [63]. The neurodevelopmental outcome associated with perinatal mother-to-child CHIKV infection will be discussed in Section 4.5.

To investigate the potential for serological evidence of congenital infection in apparently healthy neonates born to women infected with CHIKV during pregnancy, we monitored the kinetics of transplacental CHIKV-specific IgG abs within the CHIMERE cohort study [55].

There was no evidence of asymptomatic congenital CHIKV infection as the 590 participating neonates were all negative for CHIKV-specific IgM at birth and the 368 children with CHIKV-specific IgG present at birth had undetectable levels of CHIKV-specific IgG by a mean of 7.7 months (range: 1–24 months). Seroreversion time (i.e., the time needed to clear transplacental IgG from infant blood or the duration until IgG is undetectable) was inversely correlated to the timing of exposure during pregnancy. Preterm-born infants seroversed earlier. Full-term small-for-gestational age seroreversed earlier than full-term normal-for-gestational age neonates (Figure 3).

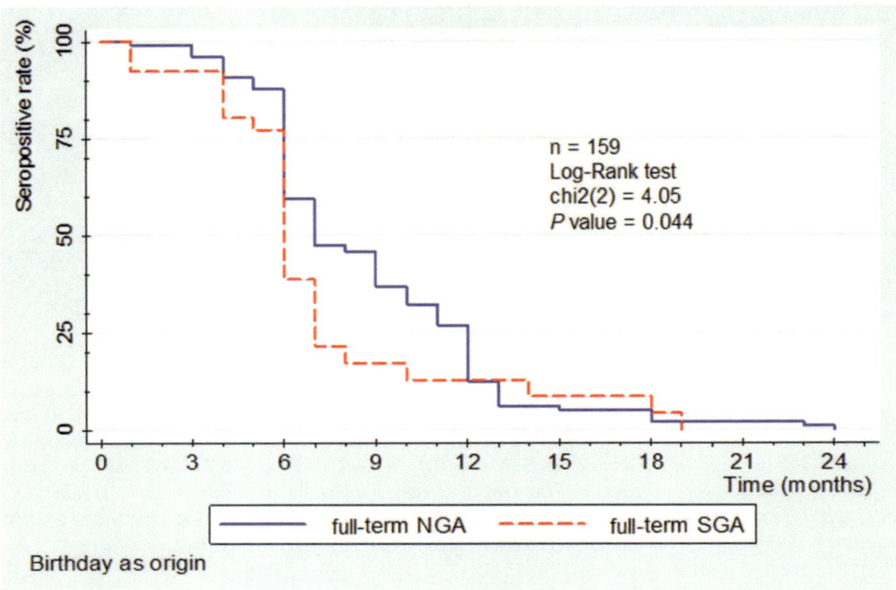

These Kaplan-Meier curves illustrate the bodysize-dependent transfer of transplacental CHIKV-specific IgG antibodies: the seropositivity rate is lower in the first post-natal year and the seroreversion time is shorter in full-term small-for-gestational age neonates compared to full-term normal-for gestational-age counterparts.

Figure 3. Seroreversion time of transplacental CHIKV-specific IgG antibodies in full-term normal-for-gestational age (NGA) and full-term small-for-gestational age (SGA) infants, CHIMERE study, Reunion island 2008 (i.e., "for more details, see [55].").

These data corroborate a time-dependent and size-dependent placental transfer of maternal IgG: the longer the period of exposure to maternal IgG and the larger the placenta, the higher the load of the IgG transferred to the fetus, and the longer the seroreversion time and theoretically the child's individual protection. These issues may be helpful for maternal or postnatal immunization, should a vaccine become available.

4.3. Chikungunya fever in infants

To the best of our knowledge, only a few case series described the clinical manifestations of postnatally acquired CF in infants [64–71].

The largest pediatric series published to date, from Kerala, India, including 357 suspected and 35 confirmed cases, reported 140 infants of whom 57% had circulatory collapse and 80% febrile seizures [66]. In another series from Kerala including 56 infants with confirmed CHIKV infection, the main symptoms were fever (100%), skin rash (100%), acrocyanosis (75%), diarrhea (41%), atypical febrile seizures (39%), irritability (26%), lethargy/poor feeding (21%), and limb edema (11%) [67]. Note that the authors have dissected the sequence of skin involvement: abrupt onset of generalized erythematous rash (day 0 to 2 of fever), maculopapular rash (day 2 to 4), vesiculobullous lesions (day 3 to 6), peeling (day 6 to 10), and hypo- or hyperpigmentation (>day 10).

These data have been confirmed in La Réunion island where half of the infants below 6 months of age exhibited vesiculobullous skin lesions [68, 88]. Importantly, besides the susceptibility for neurological complications (six-fold higher incidence rate of encephalitis) [34], these vesiculobullous skin lesions have emerged as the most characteristic finding of CHIKV infection in this age group [25, 70, 72, 73]. Severe perianal involvement is a characteristic localization [67]. Blisters sometimes cover more than 30% of the body surface, and therefore management resembles that of severe burn patients [70]. Mucosal lesions have not been reported to date. Histopathologic examination of the blisters occurring in the course of CHIKV infection reveals intraepidermal cleavage (splitting beneath and within the stratum granulosum) with CHIKV-specific IgM deposits onto the basal layer or the dermal capillaries. On follow-up, long-term repigmentation is usually observed, sometimes with skin sequelae including discrete peripheral hyperpigmentation and keloid scars.

4.4. Chikungunya fever in children

As for children in the first year of life, fever is the main symptom in older children and is usually high grade (102/39–104/40 °F/°C) of sudden onset (<24 hours) and single-spiked [25, 64, 65, 74]. Febrile seizures are common but variably present in 14-80% of the cases. They also occur beyond the typical age range of 6 months to 6 years [25, 64, 69, 73, 74]. Other common symptoms accompanying fever include musculoskeletal pain (30–50%), skin rash (>30%), headache (15%), and photophobia (<10%) [25, 68, 74].

In contrast to adults, arthritis is uncommon in children [25, 74]: 9 of 22 (40%) children reported arthralgia and 6 of 22 (27%) reported arthritis during the Vellore epidemic, Tamil Nadu, India [64]. Residual arthralgia or arthritis is also far less frequent than reported in adults. In the TELECHIK population-based cohort study [75], they were reported in ~6% of children, two years after acute infection. Unfortunately, these data cannot be retrieved from observational studies or case series, either by lack of follow-up or inability to extract the pediatric data.

The most commonly reported skin manifestations were maculopapular exanthema (morbilliform or generalized) [35, 74, 76], pigmentary changes (diffuse or macular) [77], and intertriginous aphthous-like ulcers [75]. Itching is common. Vesiculobullous skin lesions are possible but rare beyond 1 year of age [77].

Hemorrhagic manifestations including epistaxis, gum, subconjunctival bleeding, and purpura are observed in ~10% of pediatric cases [25]. They are less severe than in children dengue fever.

CHIKV-associated sepsis is less common in toddlers (1–2 years) than in infants (<1 year) and exceptional in children (3–18 years) [64, 76, 78]. In infants, circulatory collapse should prompt cardiologic investigation, including echocardiography as cases of acute cardiac failure have been described during CF [79–81] and myocarditis demonstrated in a young adult [82].

Neurological symptoms have been notified in the acute phase of CF in 25–30% of hospitalized children on the island of La Réunion [25, 68, 69, 83] but were also observed in India [64–66, 74, 84–86]. Their burden will be described in the next section.

4.5. Chikungunya-virus-associated central nervous system (CNS) disease

CHIKV has long been suspected to be a neurovirulent pathogen [86]. Thus, the seminal publications of CHIKV-associated neuropathology came from India [64] and Cambodia [87].

Among the neurological manifestations complicating CHIKV infection, three distinct clinical patterns can be seen: (i) CHIKV-associated CNS disease, namely encephalopathy of chikungunya origin and CHIKV-associated encephalitis [34, 42]; (ii) CHIKV-associated peripheral nerve disease, including myeloradiculitis and polyradiculoneuritis, and (iii) a putative nonspecific neurobiologic disease (e.g., lethargy, irritability, altered mental status, mild cognitive disorders, fatigue, etc.) not entirely satisfying the two aforementioned conditions and presumably resulting from penetration of proinflammatory cytokines through the BBB. Although nonspecific neurological symptoms and CHIKV-associated CNS disease are deemed to be common in children, CHIKV-associated peripheral nerve disease (Guillain-Barré syndrome often referred as acute flaccid paralysis) seems exceptional [74, 87].

Indeed, hospital-based series have identified headaches, seizures, altered mental status such as confusion or delirium, and neck stiffness as common signs of CNS involvement [83, 84]. Status epilepticus, complex seizures, and encephalitis are being reported as the most serious complications of CNS involvement [25]. Importantly, while the overall burden of neurological manifestations seems to increase with age, the incidence of CHIKV-associated CNS disease peaks in children less than 5 years [34]. This is also highlighted by the fact that fatigue or mild neuropsychiatric symptoms (attention difficulties, sleep, memory, or mood disorders) were reported for 84% of school-age children participating to the TELECHIK cohort study, on average 2 years after acute infection [7].

We propose to represent the burden of neurological manifestations of CF in children using a pyramid (Figure 4), as done classically in public health for vector-borne zoonosis [88].

Little is known on the long-term outcome of CHIKV-associated CNS disease [34]. For example, the neurodevelopmental outcome of perinatal mother-to-child CHIKV infection in the CHIMERE cohort study revealed that 51% of infected neonates had a global neurodevelopmental delay (GND; Brunet-Lézine development quotient ≤ 85) at the age of 2 years [56]. The skill areas affected were coordination and language (57%), sociability (36%), and movement/

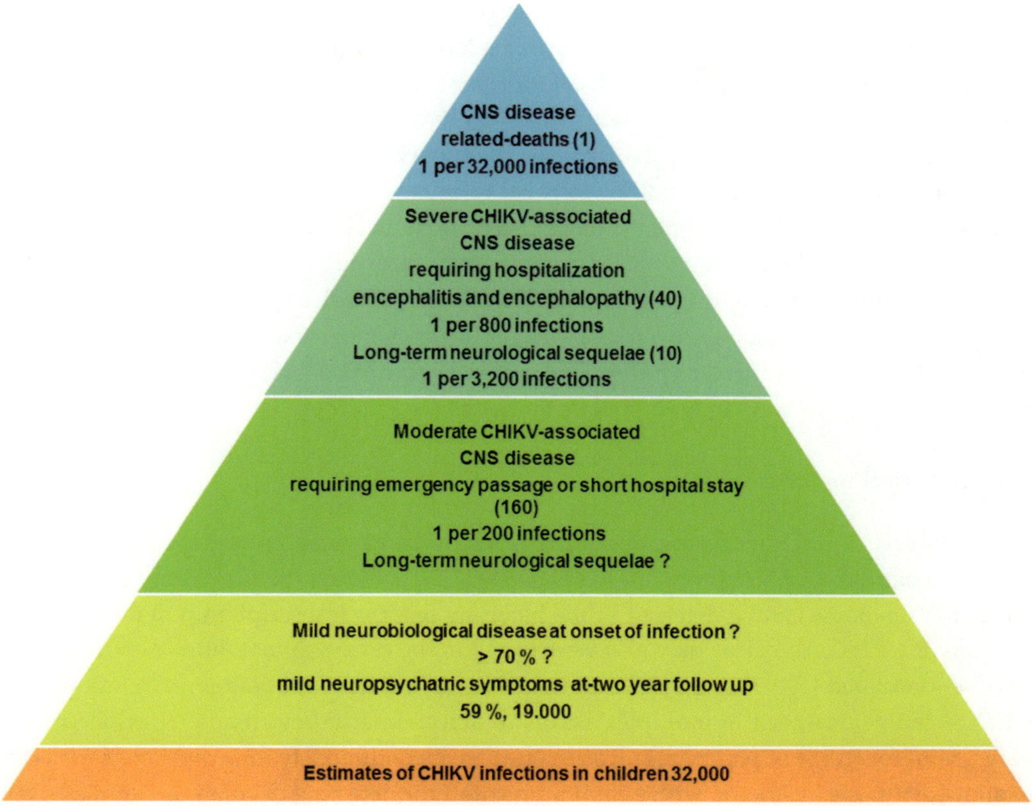

This pyramid presents the incidence data and proportions of clinical forms according to epidemiological standards for reporting the community burden of infectious diseases.

Figure 4. Burden of CHIKV-associated CNS disease in children, Southern Reunion island, 2009 (i.e., "source SERO-CHIK, TELECHIK and ENCEPHALCHIK studies, see [11, 7, 34].").

posture (27%). Importantly, CHIKV infection was an independent predictor for GND after adjustment for maternal social status, infant's weight-for-gestational age, and head circumference, but also when controlling for preterm birth and breastfeeding. Five of the 12 neonates with CHIKV-associated "encephalopathy" developed a microcephaly of whom 4 matched the definition of cerebral palsy. Note that GND was observed in 38% of the CHIKV-perinatally infected neonates in which CNS disease was not previously suspected.

5. Diagnosis

5.1. Differential diagnosis

Even though viral diseases are a major public health concern, they are not given due recognition as a cause of fever in febrile children in resource limited settings [89]. The differential diagnosis of a febrile child or pregnant woman with recent travel to or residency in tropical areas affected by CHIKV is broad and should include malaria, dengue, influenza, hepatitis, typhoid fever, leptospirosis, and rickettsial infections [25]. In addition, in areas, where these pathogens are present, infections with other alphaviruses, flaviviruses, filoviruses, and bunyaviruses should be considered. In infants, staphylococcal scalded skin syndrome [70] and Kawasaki syndrome [90] should additionally be considered and excluded as the two diagnoses require a specific treatment. Among those listed, dengue is the infection most capable of mimicking CF [25]. Clinical signs including fever pattern, arthralgia, and rash cannot reliably be used to distinguish dengue fever from CF [91]. However, rash appears earlier in the course of CF than it does in dengue fever, and dengue fever is more likely to be associated with bleeding. Pregnancy-induced hypertension, placental abruption, and preterm labor are more common in pregnant woman with dengue than with CF [51, 52].

5.2. Virological methods

After onset of CF, the viral load can rapidly reach up to 10^8 genome copies per ml of blood (even a maximum of 2.5×10^8 cps/ml in neonates) [1, 42]. During the first 5 days of infection, the CHIKV genome can be detected in the blood by reverse transcription polymerase chain reaction (RT-PCR). The virus may also be detected in the cerebrospinal fluid of children with CHIKV-associated CNS disease [25] and in blisters of infants with bullous skin lesions [62]. RT-PCR can be designed in multiplex assays to detect other arboviruses [92], which can be very useful for triage of patients [1]. Techniques have continuously improved over the years to allow diagnosis in 2 hours with a minimum cutoff for detecting circulating viremia as low as 40 genome copies/ml using a 5 ml blood sample in TaqMan real-time PCR [93].

5.3. Serological methods

CHIKV-specific IgM and IgG can be detected in serum by enzyme-like-immunosorbent assay (ELISA) immunocapture. CHIKV-specific IgM are detectable from 3 to 8 days after onset of infection (p.o.i.) and may persist for several months to up to 2 years. CHIKV-specific IgG are detectable from 4 to 10 days p.o.i. and may persist for years [1] and potentially lifelong. Although, improvement has diminished the possibility of cross-reactivity of IgG with other viruses of the Semliki antigenic serocomplex, it may still be useful to ensure a reliable diagnosis of CHIKV infection by using IgG seroconversion (increase by a factor ≥4). In areas where CHIKV and other closely related alphaviruses coexist, plaque reduction neutralization testing becomes a necessary adjunct to confirm CHIKV infection [94].

5.4. Diagnostic testing depends on timing of illness onset

The molecular assays (TaqMan real-time PCR, RT-LAMP assay, and reverse transcription PCR) are more sensitive in the early stage of CF (2–5 days p.o.i.) when CHIKV-specific IgM are not yet detectable. In the later stages of CF (>5 days p.o.i.), CHIKV-specific IgM is more sensitive than PCR. Experts recommend that ELISA IgM be used as an initial screening test

http://dx.doi.org/10.5772/64424

followed by one of the molecular assays in samples negative for IgM in the early stage of CF [95].

6. Therapeutic options

6.1. Pregnant women

There is no specific treatment for CF. CF in pregnant women should be treated with antipyretics and analgesics to prevent miscarriage, fetal demise, and limit the harmful consequences of fever, as well as this new competing risk for the neurodevelopmental outcome of preterm neonates.

6.2. Children

As in pregnant women, there is no specific treatment for CF. Management is symptomatic and focuses on adequate hydration, antipyretics, and analgesics (paracetamol/acetaminophen 60–80 mg/kg/day) [25]. Experts recommend withholding salicylates, steroidal, and nonsteroidal anti-inflammatory drugs (NSAIDs), as they may facilitate bleeding manifestations [73]. In La Réunion island, ibuprofen had been thought to precipitate infant blistering but the association was not statistically significant [96].

There are no antivirals that have been licensed to treat CF. Ribavirin and IFN-α have *in vitro* an antiviral activity against CHIKV [97], the first being able to alleviate chronic arthralgia and swelling [1]; however, neither one is recommended for use due to risk for side effects and nor the other has been tested in children. It is hoped that in the future, safe and effective antivirals will be able to offer specific CHIKV therapy.

Although persistent joint pain may be challenging to manage, NSAIDs together with corticosteroids or methotrexate successfully have been used in adults [25].

Passive immunotherapy has proven efficacious in the cure of CHIKV infections in animal models [98] and is currently being tested in neonates born to viremic mothers (i.e., "see ClinicalTrials.gov number NCT02230163") in French West Indies and French Guiana [1].

7. Prevention

7.1. Vaccination

By the end of year 2015, several promising vaccine candidates have reached late preclinical or phase-1 testing and two have been scheduled for phase-2 trials [99]. The licensure of vaccines will be challenging because of difficulties conducting affordable efficacy trials and predicting future markets [1].

7.2. Control of the vector

Preventive measures include community mobilization for eradication of breeding sites of Ae. mosquitoes [100], which primarily dwell in natural and artificial water-filled container habitats. During epidemics, peridomestic spraying of insecticides by residents and space spraying by vector controls teams are key for reducing adult mosquito populations.

7.3. Individual protection against mosquito bites

Appropriate clothing (long clothes for gardening and evening walks) may minimize skin exposure. Insect repellents containing DEET (N,N-diethyl-3-methylbenzamide), IR3535 (3-[N-acetyl-N-butyl]-aminopropionic acid ethyl ester), or picaridin (1-piperidinecarboxylic acid and 2-(2-hydroxyethyl)-1-methylpropylester) are effective [101]. DEET is safe for use in pregnancy, though it is known to cross the placenta, and can be used in children of 3 months of age and older [102]. Its putative neurotoxicity remains controversial [103]. In addition, insecticide-treated nets are important for pregnant women, infants, and children who take daytime naps. Indeed, rest under treated nets for acute patients should be considered as a pillar of community protection and in the hospital setting during the period of viremia for at least 2 weeks. The effectiveness of both types of mechanical preventive measures has not been assessed.

8. Conclusions and perspectives

CF is a tropical arthropod-borne virus infection whose geographical distribution has grown steadily over the last decade as a result of global warming and globalization of transports. CHIKV can also be transmitted vertically from mother-to-child during the perinatal period when the parturient woman is highly viremic during labor. In the pediatric population, severe forms of CF may occur, and the CNS is particularly affected with encephalitis as the major syndrome of CHIKV-associated CNS disease. At pediatric ages, neonates and small infants below 6 months of age have the highest risk for case fatality and lifelong disabilities.

Several knowledge gaps remain for CF in both pregnant women and children including: (i) the effectiveness of postponing delivery and caesarian section; (ii) the genotype-specific virulence of CHIKV and its ability to cause perinatal mother-to-child infection, CNS infection, or other life-threatening complications; and (iii) are there possible interactions between CHIKV and other circulating arboviruses in Aedes mosquito vectors susceptible to explain the rise of arbovirus-related neurological disease? This question is critical both for CHIKV and Zika virus, a conqueror flavivirus which has supplanted CHIKV wherever it has tried to establish in recent years; (iv) the subtle long-term morbidities that CF may cause in children. The absence of autopsy data with reliable histopathological findings (immunochemistry staining) prevents understanding of the human CNS neuropathology.

Benchmarking of observational studies, meta-analysis of individual patient data, and well-designed clinical trials should be of paramount importance to address these knowledge gaps.

Future antivirals and vaccines may alleviate some of the disease burden, but for now vector control and human personal protection are the only means of CF prevention.

Author details

Patrick Gérardin[1,2,3*], A. Désirée LaBeaud[4], Nicole Ritz[5,6] and Xavier Fritel[7,8]

*Address all correspondence to: patrick.gerardin@chu-reunion.fr

1 CHU Réunion, Saint-Pierre, Reunion, France

2 Inserm Centre for Clinical Investigation (CIC 1410), Saint-Pierre, Reunion, France

3 Université de La Réunion, CNRS 9192, INSERM U1187, IRD 249, CHU de La Réunion, Unité Mixte Processus Infectieux en Milieu Insulaire Tropical (PIMIT), Plateforme Technologique CYROI, Sainte-Clotilde, La Réunion, France

4 Stanford School of Medicine, Palo Alto, CA, USA

5 Infectious Diseases Unit and Paediatric Pharmacology, University Children's Hospital Basel, The University of Basel, Switzerland

6 The Royal Children's Hospital Melbourne, The University of Melbourne, Parkville, Australia

7 Department of Gynecology and Obstetrics, CHU Poitiers, France

8 Inserm Centre for Clinical Investigation (CIC1402), Poitiers, France

References

[1] Weaver SC, Lecuit M. Chikungunya virus and the global spread of a mosquito-borne disease. New Engl J Med 2015; 372: 1231–1239. doi: 10.1056/NEJMra1406035.

[2] Lumsden WHR. An epidemic of virus disease in southern province, Tanganyika territory, in 1952–53. II. General description and epidemiology. Trans R Soc Trop Med Hyg 1955; 49: 33–57. doi: 10.1016/0035-9203(55)90081-X.

[3] Ross RW. The newala epidemic. III. The virus: isolation, pathogenic properties and relationship to the epidemic. J Hyg (London) 1956; 54: 177–191. doi: 10.1017/S0022172400044442.

[4] Robinson MC. I. Clinical features. An epidemic virus disease in southern province, Tanganyika territory in 1952–53. Trans R Soc Trop Med Hyg 1955; 49: 28–32. doi: 10.1016/0035-9203(55)90080-8.

[5] Borgherini G, Poubeau P, Staikowsky F, et al. Outbreak of chikungunya on Reunion island: early clinical and laboratory features in 157 adult patients. Clin Infect Dis 2007; 44: 1401–1407. doi: 10.1086/517537.

[6] Labeaud AD, Bashir F, King CH. Measuring the burden of arboviral diseases: the spectrum of morbidity and mortality from four prevalent infections. Popul Health Metrics. 2011; 9: 1. doi: 10.1186/1478-7954-9-1.

[7] Gérardin P, Fianu A, Malvy D, et al. Perceived morbidity and community burden after a chikungunya outbreak: the TELECHIK survey, a population-based cohort study. BMC Med 2011; 9: 5. doi: 10.1186/1741-7015-9-5.

[8] Mathew AJ, Goyal V, Gorge E, et al. Rheumatic musculoskeletal pain and disorders in a naïve group of individual 15 months following a chikungunya viral epidemic in South India: population based study. Int J Clin Pract 2011; 65: 1306–1312. doi: 10.1111/j.1742-1241.2011.02792.x.

[9] Rodriguez-Morales AJ, Cardona-Ospina JA, Villamil-Gomez W, Paniz-Mondolfi AE. How many patients with post-chikungunya chronic inflammatory rheumatism can we expect in the new endemic areas of Latin America ? Rheumatol Int 2015; 35: 2091–2094. doi: 10.1007/s00296-015-3302-5.

[10] Renault P, Solet JL, Sissoko D, et al. A major epidemic of chikungunya virus in Reunion island, France, 2005–2006. Am J Trop Med Hyg 2007; 77: 727–731.

[11] Gérardin P, Guernier V, Perrau J, et al. Estimating chikungunya prevalence in La Reunion island outbreak by serosurveys: two methods for two critical times of the epidemic. BMC Infect Dis 2008; 8: 99. doi: 10.1186/1471-2334-8-99.

[12] Economopoulou A, Dominguez M, Helynck B, et al. Atypical chikungunya virus infections: clinical manifestations, mortality and risk factors for severe disease during the 2005–2006 outbreak on Réunion. Epidemiol Infect 2008; 137: 534–541. doi: 10.1017/S0950268808001167.

[13] Lemant J, Boisson V, Winer A, et al. Serious acute chikungunya virus infection requiring intensive care during the Reunion island outbreak in 2005–2006. Crit Care Med 2008; 36: 2536–2541. doi: 10.1097/CCM.0b013e318183f2d2.

[14] Josseran L, Paquet C, Zehgoun A, et al. Chikungunya disease outbreak, Reunion island outbreak, Emerg Infect Dis 2006; 12: 1994–1995. doi: 10.3201/eid1212.060710.

[15] Mavalankar D, Shastri P, Bandyopadhyay T, Parmar J, Ramani KV. Increased mortality rate associated with chikungunya epidemic, Ahmedabad, India. Emerg Infect Dis 2008; 14: 412–415. doi: 10.3201/eid1403.070720.

[16] Fischer M, Staples JE. Notes from the field: chikungunya virus spreads in the Americas - Caribbean and South America, 2013–2014. MMWR Morb Mortal Wkly Rep 2014; 63: 500–501.

[17] Sharp TM, Shieh WS, Levine R, et al. Clinicopathologic characteristics and immunocolocalization of viral antigens in chikungunya-associated fatal cases—Puerto Rico, 2014. In: Proceedings of the ID Week 2015 Conference, October 7–11; San Diego. Oral abstract session, talk 1975. Available from: http://idsa.confex.com/idsa/2015/webprogram/Paper51373.html.

[18] Volk SM, Chen R, Tsetsarkin KA, et al. Genome-scale phylogenetic analysis of chikungunya virus reveal independent ermergences of recent epidemics and various evolutionary rates. J Virol 2010; 84: 6497–6504. doi: 10.1128/JVI.01603-09.

[19] Carey DE. Chikungunya and dengue: a case of mistaken identity? J Hist Med Allied Sci 1971: 26: 243–262. doi: 10.1093/jhmas/XXVI.3.243.

[20] Paupy C, Delatte H, Bagny L, Corbel V, Fontenille D. Aedes albopictus. An arbovirus vector: from the darkness to the light. Microbes Infect 2009; 11: 1177–1185. doi: 10.1016/j.micinf.2009.05.005.

[21] Reiter P, Fontenille D, Paupy C. Aedes albopictus as an epidemic vector od chikungunya virus: another emerging problem? Lancet Infect Dis 2006; 6: 463–464. doi : 10.1016/S1473-3099(06)70531-X.

[22] Tsetsarkin KA, Chen R, Yun R, et alMulti-peaked adaptive landscape for chikungunya virus evolution predicts continued fitness optimization in Aedes albopictus mosquitoes. Nat Comm 2014; 5: 4084. doi: 10.1038/ncomms5084.

[23] Leparc-Goffart I, Nougairede A, Cassadou S, Prat C, de Lamballerie X. Chikungunya in the Americas. Lancet 2014; 383: 514. doi: 10.1016/S0140-6736(14)60185-9.

[24] Pan American Health Organization. Number of reported cases of chikungunya fever in the Americas—epidemiological week 46 (November 20, 2015 [cited 2015 Nov 21]). Available from: http://paho.org/hg/index.php?option com docman&task=doc download&Itemid=270&gid=32304&lang=en.

[25] Ritz N, Hüfnagel M, Gérardin P. Chikungunya in children. Pediatr Infect Dis J 2015; 34:789–791. doi: 10.1097/INF.0000000000000716.

[26] Voss JE, Vaney MV, Duquerroy S, et al. Glycoprotein organization of chikungunya virus particles revealed by X-ray crystallography. Nature 2010; 468: 709–712. doi: 10.1038/nature09555.

[27] Tsetsarkin KA, Vanlandingam DL, McGee CE, Higgs S. A single mutation in chikungunya virus affects vector specificity and epidemic potential. PLoS Pathog 2007; 3: e201. doi: 10.1371/journal.ppat.0030201.

[28] Diallo M, Thonnon J, Traoré-Lamizana M, Fontenille D. Vectors of chikungunya virus in Senegal. Am J Trop Med Hyg 1999; 60: 281–286.

[29] Gérardin P. Aspects pédiatriques de la dengue et du chikungunya. Arch Pediatr 2010: 17: 86–90. doi: 10.1016/j.arcped.2009.09.001.

[30] Dubrulle M, Mousson L, Moutailler S, Vazeille M, Failloux AB. Chikungunya virus and Aedes mosquitoes: saliva is infectious as soon as two days after oral infection. PLoS One 2009; 4: e5895. doi: 10.1371/journal.pone.0005895.

[31] Gasque P, Couderc T, Lecuit M, Roques P, Ng LF. Chikungunya virus pathogenesis and immunity. Vector Borne Zoonotic Dis 2015; 15: 241–249. doi: 10.1089/vbz.2014.1710.

[32] Teng TS, Kam YW, Lee B, et al. A systematic meta-analysis of immune signatures in patients with acute chikungunya virus infections. J Infect Dis 2015; 211: 1925–1935. doi: 10.1093/infdis/jiv049.

[33] Couderc T, Chrétien F, Schilte C, et al. A mouse model for chikungunya: young age and inefficient type-I interferon signaling are risk factors for severe disease. PLoS Pathog 2008; 4: e29. doi: 10.1371/journal.ppat.0040029.

[34] Gérardin P, Couderc T, Bintner M, et al. Chikungunya virus-associated encephalitis: acohortstudy on La Réunion island, 2005–2009. Neurology 2016; 86: 94–102. [Epubahead of print 2015 Nov 25]. doi: 10.1212/WNL.0000000000002234.

[35] Inamadar AC, Palit A, Sampagavi VV, Raghunath S, Deshmukh NS. Cutaneous manifestations of chikungunya fever: observations made during a recent outbreak in south India. Int J Dermatol 2008; 47: 154–159. doi: 10.1111/j.1365-4632.2008.03478.x.

[36] Lum FM, Teo TH, Lee WM, Kam YW, Renia L, Ng LF. An essential role of antibodies in the control of chikungunya virus infection. J Immunol 2013; 190: 6295–6302. doi: 10.4049/jimmunol.1300304.

[37] Her Z, Malleret B, Chang M, et al. Active infection of human blood monocytes by chikungunya virus triggers an innate immune response. J Immunol 2010; 184: 5903–5913. doi: 10.4049/jimmunol.0904181.

[38] Hoarau JJ, Jaffar-Bandjee MC, Krejbich-Trotot P, et al. Persistent chronic inflammation and infection by chikungunya arthritogenic alphavirus in spite of robust host immune response. J Immunol 2010; 184: 5914–5927. doi: 10.4049/jimmunol.0900255.

[39] Saito S, Sakaï M. Th1/Th2 balance in preeclampsia. J Reprod Immunol 2003; 59: 161–173. doi: 10.1016/S0165-0378(03)00045-7.

[40] Ceccaldi PF, Longuet P, Mandelbrot L. Infections virales émergentes et grossesse. Gynecol Obstet Fertil 2007; 35: 339–342. doi : 10.1016/j.gyobfe.2007.02.020.

[41] Lenglet Y, Barau G, Robillard PY, et al. Infection à Chikungunya chez la femme enceinte et risque de transmission materno-foetale. Etude dans un contexte d'épidémie en

2005–2006 à l'île de La Réunion. J Gynecol Ostet Biol Reprod (Paris) 2006; 35: 578–583. doi: JGYN-10-2006-35-6-0368-2315-101019-200605061.

[42] Gérardin P, Barau G, Michault A, et al. Multidisciplinary prospective study of mother-to-child chikungunya virus infections on the island of La Réunion. PLoS Med 2008; 5: e60. doi: 10.1371/journal.pmed.0050060.

[43] Fritel X, Rollot O, Gérardin P, et al. Chikungunya virus infection during pregnancy, Reunion, France, 2006. Emerg Infect Dis. 2010; 16: 418–425. doi: 10.3201/eid1603.091403.

[44] Fritel X, Catteau C, Calliez F, Brodel A, Vaillant JL, Ansquin H. Chikungunya outbreak, pregnancy outcome and perinatal mortality: observational study about 40,000 pregnancies and deliveries on Réunionisland, during 2004–2006. In: Proceedings of the 13th International Congress on Infectious Disease, 2008 June 19–22, Kuala Lumpur. Abstract published in: Int J Infect Dis 2008; 12 (Suppl 1): e328. doi:10.1016/j.ijid.2008.05.880.

[45] Touret Y, Randrianaivo H, Michault A, et al. Early maternal-fetal transmission of the chikungunya virus. Presse Med 2006; 35: 1656–1658. doi: PM-11-2006-35-11-0755-4982-101019-200608661.

[46] Her Z, Teng TS, Tan JL, et al. Loss of TLR3 aggravates CHIKV replication and pathology due to an altered-virus specific neutralizing response. Embo Mol Med 2014; 7: 24–41. doi: 10.15252/emmm.201404459.

[47] Zhang J, H Wei, D Wu, Tian Z. Toll-like receptor 3 agonist induces impairment of uterine vascular remodeling and fetal losses in CBA ◎ DBA/ 2 mice. J Reprod Immunol 2007; 74: 61–67. doi : 10.1016/j.jri.2006.10.005.

[48] Chen CI, Clark DC, Pesaveto P, et al. Comparative pathogenesis of epidemic and enzootic chikungunya viruses in pregnant Rhesus macaque model. Am J Trop Med Hyg 2010; 83: 1249–1258. doi: 10.4269/ajtmh.2010.10-0290.

[49] Nair PMC. Chikungunya in neonates. Indian Pediatr 2008; 45: 605.

[50] Gérardin P, Rollot O, Touret Y, et al. Infection à virus chikungunya pendant la grossesse : pas de relation entre le moment de l'exposition et le poids de naissance. Etude exposé-non exposé. Bull Soc Pathol Exot 2007; 108: 353–354. doi: 10.13140/RG.2.1.1200.5847.

[51] Basurko C, Carles G, Youssef M, Guindi WE. Maternal and fetal consequences of dengue during pregnancy. Eur J Obstet Gynecol Reprod Biol 2009; 147: 29–32. doi: 10.1016/j.ejogrb.2009.06.028.

[52] Friedmann EE, Dallah F, Harville EW, et al. Symptomatic dengue infection during pregnancy and infant outcomes: a retrospective cohort study. PLoS Negl Trop Dis 2014; 8: e3226. doi: 10.1371/journal.pntd.0003226.

[53] Robillard PY, Boumahni B, Gérardin P, et al. Transmission verticale materno-foetale du virus chikungunya. Presse Med 2006; 35: 785–788. doi:10.1016/S0755-4982(06)74690-5.

[54] Ramful D, Carbonnier M, Pasquet M, et al. Mother-to-child transmission of chikungunya virus infection. Pediatr Infect Dis J 2007; 26: 811–815. doi: 10.1097/INF.0b013e3180616d4f.

[55] Ramful D, Sampériz S, Fritel X, et al. Antibody kinetics in infants exposed to chikungunya virus infection during pregnancy reveals absence of congenital Infection. J Infect Dis 2014; 209: 1726–1730. doi: 10.1093/infdis/jit814.

[56] Gérardin P, Samperiz S, Ramful D, et al. Neurocognitive outcome of children exposed to perinatal mother-to-child chikungunya virus infection: the CHIMERE cohort study on Reunion Island. PLoS Negl Trop Dis. 2014;8: e2996. doi: 10.1371/journal.pntd.0002996.

[57] Passi GR, Khan YS, Chitnis DS. Chikungunya in neonates. Indian Pediatr 2008; 45: 240–242.

[58] Shrivastava A, Beg MW, Gujrati C, Gopalan N, Rao PVL. Management of a vertically transmitted neonatal chikungunya thrombocytopenia. Indian J Pediatr 2011: 78: 1008–1009. doi: 10.1007/s12098-011-0371-7.

[59] Gopakumar H, Ramachandran S. Congenital chikungunya. J Clin Neonatol 2012; 1: 155–156. doi: 10.4103/2249-4847.101704.

[60] Vasani RV, Kanhere S, Chaudahri K, et al. Congenital chikungunya—a cause of neonatal hyperpigmentation. Pediatr Dermatol 2015 Jul 23 [Epub ahead of print]. doi: 10.1111/pde.12650.

[61] Villamil-Gomez W, Alba-Silvera L, Menco-Ramos A, et al. Congenital chikungunya virus infection in Sincelejo, Colombia: a case series. J Trop Pediatr 2015; 61: 386–392. doi: 10.1093/tropej/fmv051.

[62] Le Bomin A, Hebert JC, Marty P, Delaunay P. Chikungunya confirmé chez l'enfant à Mayotte à propos de 50 cas hospitalisés février-juin 2006. Med Trop (Mars) 2008; 68: 491–495.

[63] Shenoy S, Pradeep GCM. Neurodevelopmental outcome of neonates with vertically transmitted chikungunya fever. Indian Pediatr 2012; 49: 238–240.

[64] Jadhav M, Namboodripad M, Carman RH, Carey DE, Myer RM. Chikungunya disease in infants and children in Vellore: a report of clinical and haematological features of virologically proved cases. Indian J Med Res 1965; 53: 764–776.

[65] Thiruvengadam KV, Kalyanasundaram V, Rajkopal J. Clinical and pathological studies on chikinungunya fever in Madras city. Indian J Med Res 1965; 53: 729–744.

[66] Elenjickal MG, Sushamabai S. Outbreak of Chikungunya disease in Kerala in 2007. Indian Pediatr 2009; 46: 440–441.

[67] Valamparampil JJ, Chirakkarot S, Letha S, Jayakumar C, Gopinathan KM. Clinical profile of chikungunya in infants. Indian J Pediatr 2009; 76: 151–155. doi: 10.1007/s12098-009-0045-x.

[68] Ernould S, Walters H, Alessandri JL, et al.Aspects pédiatriques de l'épidémie de Chikungunya à l'île de la Réunion. Arch Pediatr. 2008; 15: 253–262. doi: 10.1016/j.arcped.2007.10.019.

[69] Houdon L, Bro C, Bangui A, et al. Formes pédiatriques du Chikungunya chez 253 nourrissons et enfants hospitalisés dans le serivce de pédiatrie du Groupe Hospitalier Sud Réunion.Bull Soc Pathol Exot 2007; 100: 354–355. doi: 10.13140/RG.2.1.1092.2328.

[70] Robin S, Ramful D, Zettor J, et al. Severe bullous skin lesions associated with chikungunya virus infection in small infants. Eur J Pediatr 2010; 169: 67–72. doi: 10.1007/s00431-009-0986-0.

[71] Gupta D, Bose A, Rose W. Acquired neonatal chikungunya encephalopathy. Indian J Pediatr 2015; 82: 1065–1066. doi: 10.1007/s12098-015-1751-1.

[72] Pakran J, George M, Riyaz N, et al. Purpuric macules with vesiculobullous lesions: a novel manifestation of chikungunya. Int J Dermatol 2011; 50: 61–69. doi: 10.1111/j.1365-4632.2010.04644.x.

[73] Khandelwal K, Aara N, Ghiya BC, Bumb RA, Satoskar AR. Centro-facial pigmentation in asymptomatic chikgununya virus manifestation. J Paediatr Child Health 2012; 48: 540–544. doi: 10.1111/j.1440-1754.2012.02484.x.

[74] Sebastian MR, Lodha R, Kabra SK. Chikungunya infection in children. Indian J Pediatr 2009; 76: 185–189. doi: 10.1007/s12098-009-0049-6.

[75] Gérardin P, Fianu A, Michault A, et al. Predictors of chikungunya rheumatism: a prognostic survey ancillary to the TELECHIK cohort study. Arthritis Res Ther 2013; 15: R9. doi: 10.1186/ar4137.

[76] Haas H, Robin S, Ramful D, Houdon L, Minodier P, Gérardin P. Infections à virus Chikungunya chez l'enfant. Arch Pediatr 2009; 16 (Suppl 2): S72–S79. doi: 10.1016/S0929-693X(09)75305-9.

[77] Seetharam KA, Sridevi K, Vidyasagar P. Cutaneous manifestations of chikungunya fever. Indian Pediatr 2012; 49: 51–53.

[78] Pellot AS, Alessandri JL, Robin S, et al. Formes sévères d'infections à virus Chikungunya en réanimation pédiatrique à l'île de La Réunion. Med Trop (Mars) 2012; 72 Spec No: 88–93.

[79] Obeyesekere I, Hermon Y. Arbovirus heart disease: myocarditis and cardiomyopathy following dengue and chikungunya fever—A follow-up study. Am Heart J 1973; 85: 186–194. doi:10.1016/0002-8703(73)90459-6.

[80] Menon PR, Krishnan C, Sankar J, Gopinathan KM, Mohan G. A child with serious chikungunya virus (CHIKV) infection requiring intensive care, after an outbreak. Indian J Pediatr 2010; 77: 1326–1328. doi: 10.1007/s12098-010-0174-2.

[81] Selly JB, Boumahni B, Edmar A, et al. Dysfonction cardiaque du noeud sinusal due à une nouvelle mutation du gène SCN5A. Arch Pediatr 2012; 19: 837–841. doi: 10.1016/j.arcped.2012.04.017.

[82] Mirabel M, Vignaux O, Lebon P, Legmann P, Weber S, Meune C. Acute myocarditis due to chikungunya-virus assessed by contrast-enhanced MRI. Int J Cardiol 2007; 121: e7–e8. doi: 10.1016/j.ijcard.2007.04.153.

[83] Robin S, Ramful D, Le Seach F, et al. Neurologic manifestations of pediatric chikungunya infection. J Child Neurol 2008; 23: 1028–1035. doi: 10.1177/0883073808314151.

[84] Chandak NH, Kashyap RS, Kabra D, et al. Neurology India 2009; 57: 177–180. doi: 10.4103/0028-3886.51289.

[85] Lewthwaite P, Vasanthapuram R, Osborne JC, et al. Chikungunya virus and central nervous system infections in children, India. Emerg Infect Dis 2009; 15: 329–331. doi: 10.3201/eid1502.080902.

[86] Das T, Jaffar-Bandjee MC, Hoarau JJ, et al. Chikungunya fever: CNS infection and pathologies of a re-emerging arbovirus. Prog Neurobiol 2010; 91: 121–129. doi: 10.1016/j.pneurobio.2009.12.006.

[87] Chastel C. Infections humaines au Cambodge par le virus du Chikungunya ou un agent étroitement apparenté. II. Anatomie pathologie expérimentale. Bull Soc Patho Exot 1963; 56: 915–924.

[88] Braks M, Medlock JM, Hubalek Z, et al. Vector-borne disease intelligence: strategies to deal with disease burden and threats. Front Public Health 2014; 2: 1–11. doi: 10.3389/fpubh.2014.00280.

[89] Chipwaza B, Mugasa JP, Selemani M, et al. Dengue and chikungunya fever among viral diseases in outpatient febrile children in Kilosa district hospital, Tanzania. PLoS Negl Trop Dis 2014; 8: e3335. doi: 10.1371/journal.pntd.0003335.

[90] Lee YS, Quek Q, Koay ESC, Tang JWT. Chikungunya mimicking atypical Kawasaki disease in an infant. Pediatr Infect Dis J 2010; 29: 275–277. doi: 10.1097/INF.0b013e3181bce34d.

[91] Laoprasopwattana K, Kaewjungwad L, Jarumanokul R, Geater A. Differential diagnosis of chikungunya, dengue viral infection and other acute febrile illnesses in children. Pediatr Infect Dis J 2012; 31: 459–463. doi: 10.1097/INF.0b013e31824bb06d.

[92] Laurent P, Le Roux K, Grivard P, et al. Development of a sensitive real-time reverse transcriptase PCR assay with an internal control to detect and quantify chikungunya virus. Clin Chem 2007; 53: 1408–1414. doi: 10.1373/clinchem.2007.086595.

[93] Naze F, Le Roux K, Schuffenecker I, et al. Simultaneous detection an quantification of chikungunya, dengue, and West Nile viruses by a multiplex RT-PCR assays and dengue virys typing using high resolution melting. J Virol Methods 2009; 162: 1–7. doi: 10.1016/j.jviromet.2009.03.006.

[94] LaBeaud AD, Banda T, Brichard J, et al. High rates of o'nyongnyong and chikungunya virus transmission in coastal Kenya. PLoS Negl Trop Dis 2015; 9: e0003436. doi: 10.1371/journal.pntd.0003436.

[95] Reddy V, Ravi A, Desai A, Parida M, Powers AM, Johnson BW. Utility of IgM ELISA, TaqMan real-time RT-PCR, reverse transcription PCR, and RT-LAMP assay for the diagnosis of chikungunya fever. J Med Virol 2012; 84: 1771–1778. doi: 10.1002/jmv.23406.

[96] Herbin G, Houdon-N'Guyen L, Gérardin P, et al. Absence de relation entre prise d'ibuprofène et dermatose bulleuse chez les enfants atteints de Chikungunya? Bull Soc Pathol Exot 2006; 2: 140. doi: 10.13140/RG.2.1.1880.0082.

[97] Abnelnabi R, Neyts R, Delang L. Towards antivirals against chikungunya virus. Antiviral Res 2015; 121: 59–68. doi: 10.1016/j.antiviral.2015.06.017.

[98] Couderc T, Khandouni N, Grandadam M, et al. Prophylaxis and therapy for chikungunya virus infection. J Infect Dis 2009; 200: 516–523. doi: 10.1086/600381.

[99] Schwameis M, Buchtele N, Wadowski PP, Schoergenhofer C, Jilma B. Chikungunya vaccines in development. Hum Vaccin Immunother. 2015 Nov 10:0. [Epubahead of print]doi: 10.1080/21645515.2015.1101197.

[100] Tamburro M, Depertat T. Mesures de protection contre les moustiques à La Réunion durant l'épidémie de Chikungunya en 2005–2006. Arch Pediatr 2009; 16: 763–765. doi: 10.1016/S0929-693X(09)74143-0.

[101] Sorge F. Prévention par insectifuge chez l'enfant. Arch Pediatr 2009; 16 (Suppl 2): S115–S122. doi: 10.1016/S0929-693X(09)75313-8.

[102] Nasci RS, Wirtz RA, Brogdon WG. Protection against mosquitoes, ticks, and other arthropods. CDC Centers for Disease Control and Prevention. Available from: http://wwwnc.cdc.gov/travel/yellowbook/2016/the-pre-travel-consultation/protection-against-mosquitoes-ticks-other-arthropods.

[103] Auvin S. Neurotoxicity des répulsifs chez l'enfant: état des connaissances. Arch Pediatr 2009; 16 (Suppl 2): S769–S770. doi: 10.1016/S0929-693X(09)74145-4.

Chapter 3

Imported Cases in Continental Chile and Autochthonous In Easter Island

Cecilia Perret P.

Additional information is available at the end of the chapter

http://dx.doi.org/10.5772/63996

Abstract

Aedes aegypti is the main vector for several arboviruses including dengue, chikungunya and Zika virus. The emergence of these viruses' transmission is possible in places where the vector exists. In Chile, *A. aegypti* was introduced in the year 2000 to Easter Island, being the responsible of the first dengue outbreak by dengue 1 serotype in the country in 2002. Just recently April 2016 *Aedes aegypti* has been found in Arica, the northernmost city of the country. On Easter Island, at the beginning of 2014, Zika outbreak was diagnosed with about 170 cases reported.

The introduction of dengue and Zika virus on Easter Island was preceded by an outbreak of DEN-1 and Zika virus on the French Polynesia in 2001 and 2013, respectively. Considering the presence of chikungunya outbreak on the French Polynesia the risk of introduction of Chikungunya on Easter Island is very high.

Cases of chikungunya in continental Chile correspond to imported cases in travelers.

This chapter reviews the epidemiology and clinical features of chikungunya infection in travelers to Latin American countries and updates the situation of the risk of introduction to Easter Island.

Keywords: Chikungunya, Chile, Easter Island, travelers, autochthonous cases

1. Introduction

Aedes aegypti is the main vector for several arboviruses including dengue, chikungunya and Zika viruses. The emergence of these diseases is possible in places where the vector exists. In Chile, *A. aegypti* was introduced in the year 2000 to Easter Island with the consequent risk of the introduction of arboviral infection to its inhabitants. *Aedes aegypti* has been just introduced into Arica, the northernmost city of the country.

This chapter reviews the epidemiology and clinical features of chikungunya infection in Chilean travelers to Latin American countries and updates the situation on Easter Island and the potential risk of introduction of this infection to Chilean insular territory.

2. Epidemiological situation in Chile

2.1. Epidemiological situation in Continental Chile

Continental Chile just recently, 2016, have the presence of *Aedes aegypti* in the northernmost city of the country, but arbovirus infections are only seen in travelers to endemic areas or residents of Easter Island.

Continental Chile is surrounded by countries where the presence of *Aedes* mosquitoes is spread as it is the circulation of arboviruses, mainly dengue, and since 2014, Latin America has suffered outbreaks of chikungunya and nowadays Zika viruses. Chile was until recently the only Latin American country where there was no vector, with the exception of its insular territory, Easter Island. For this reason the Ministry of Health is continuously watching for diseases transmitted by mosquitoes as well as for the emergence of vectors by placing ovitraps and larval traps from the North of Chile to the metropolitan region (center of the country).

The study of the samples captured in these traps, received from mainland Chile and Easter Island, has shown to date presence of *Aedes* on Easter Island and in the north of Chile along with the presence of *Anopheles* [1].

Arboviral disease surveillance system has dengue as notifiable disease but not chikungunya. After the introduction of chikungunya into the Americas, in Chile 30 cases of imported chikungunya have been reported up to epidemiological week 15 of 2016, 21 in mainland Chile and 3 on Easter Island. During 2014 22 cases were reported and 6 cases during 2015. During 2016 two cases of imported chikungunya have been reported. However, chikungunya is not a notifiable disease so it is very likely that there is an underreporting of cases. In the report from the Chilean Ministry of Health, most of the cases of chikungunya in Chile came from Dominican Republic, Haiti and Bolivia. (not available online)

2.2. Chikungunya in international travelers

During 2014–2015 in the laboratory of Virology of the School of Medicine of the Pontificia Universidad Católica de Chile, we diagnosed 26 people with chikungunya infection by indirect immunofluorescence assay IgM or IgG. We obtained demographic and clinical data in 16 of them. In 4 of them the diagnosis was retrospective by IgG because they were working as voluntary corps for the Chilean Army in Haiti and they could not confirm the diagnosis until they were back several months later.

Most of them acquired the disease in Latin America and only 3 in Asia and Oceania. Countries with higher frequency of exposure were Colombia and Haiti.

Most were women (75%), average age 39 years (27–52 years old) and median-length trip was 10 days. Twelve people started to show symptoms with a median of 5 days prior to the return and 4 started to show symptoms 2.5 days on average from return. First symptom was joint pain in 69%. Arthralgia was present in 94%, arthritis in 75% and exanthema in 63%, which was itchy in the majority of cases. The median duration of arthralgia was 3 months. In the hemogram the hematocrit was normal and WBC count was 5549 cells/mm ^{3} on average with predominance of PMN and lymphopenia. The absolute count of lymphocytes in average was 1049 cells/mm^3. Only one patient presented less than 150,000 platelets/mm^3 (Table 1; unpublished data)

Symptoms	Number n=16	Percentage (%)
Myalgia	16	100
Fever	15	94
Arthralgia	15	94
Headache	13	81
Arthritis	12	75
Anorexia	12	75
Diffuse rash	10	63
Retro-orbital pain	8	50
Nauseas	7	44
Vomiting	4	25
Diarrhea	3	19
Itching	1	19

Table 1. Symptoms of 16 imported cases of confirmed chikungunya in travelers

2.3. Current situation on Easter Island

Easter Island received thousands of visitors yearly, arriving either from Santiago Airport or from Tahiti. In this territory there is a surveillance of febrile patients as well as vector surveillance to timely diagnose the introduction of any *Aedes*-borne infection due to the presence of this vector on the Island. *A. aegypti* was first noticed on the island in 2000. In 2002 a big outbreak of DEN-1 infection occurred, affecting nearly the whole island population. Only not complicated dengue cases were observed [2]. Genetic studies show that the virus was introduced from the French Polynesia [3]. Since then, sporadic cases of dengue fever have been reported. In the year 2014 occurred an outbreak of Zika infection with about 170 autochthonous cases reported being introduced again from the French Polynesia; 51 of them were confirmed by PCR at the National Institute of Public Health. Phylogenetic analysis has shown that viral strains from Easter Island were found to be most closely related to those found in the French

Polynesia (Figure 1) [4]. After the introduction of Zika virus to Brazil and its spread to Latin America during 2015 and 2016, no autochthonous cases of Zika have been diagnosed so far.

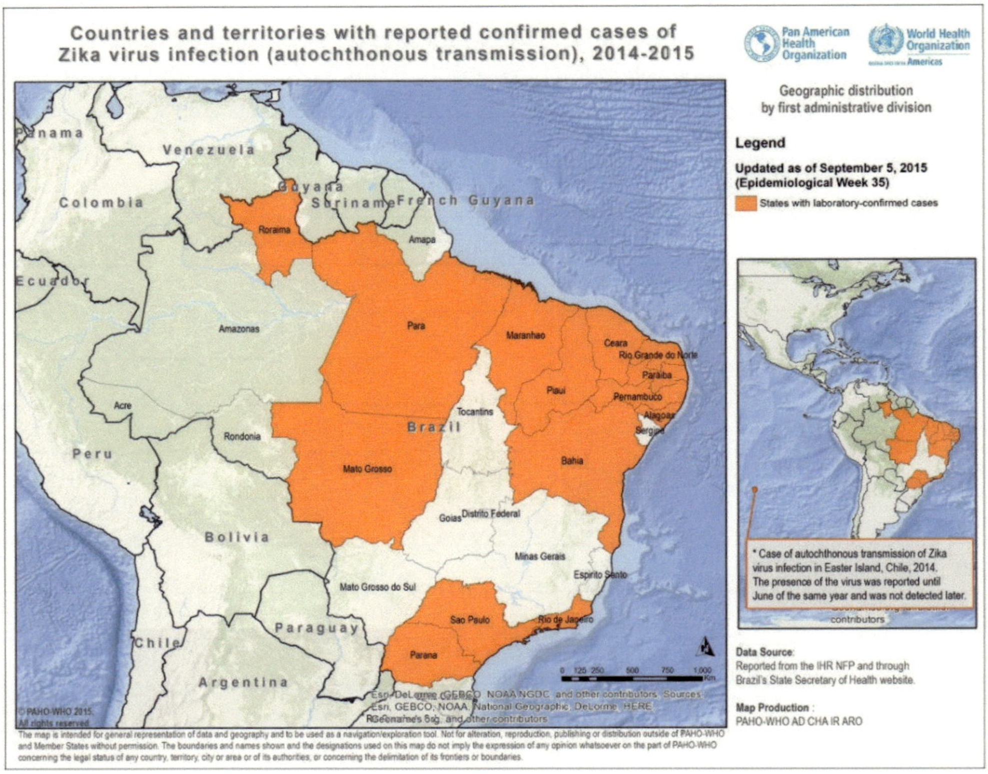

Figure 1. Countries and territories with reported confirmed cases of Zika virus infection (autochthonous transmission), 2014–2015.

A current outbreak of dengue 1 virus is occurring on the Island. Twenty nine autochthonous cases have been notified. There were no cases of severe dengue probably because of the same serotype circulating since 2002.

To date no indigenous cases of chikungunya have been reported beside 3 cases imported from Tahiti, at the beginning of 2015 and fortunately without secondary cases.

3. Conclusions

Chikungunya infection is introduced in the Americas at the end of the year 2013, in a region where the presence of its vector, *A. aegypti* and *A. albop*ictus, is highly spread. As expected in

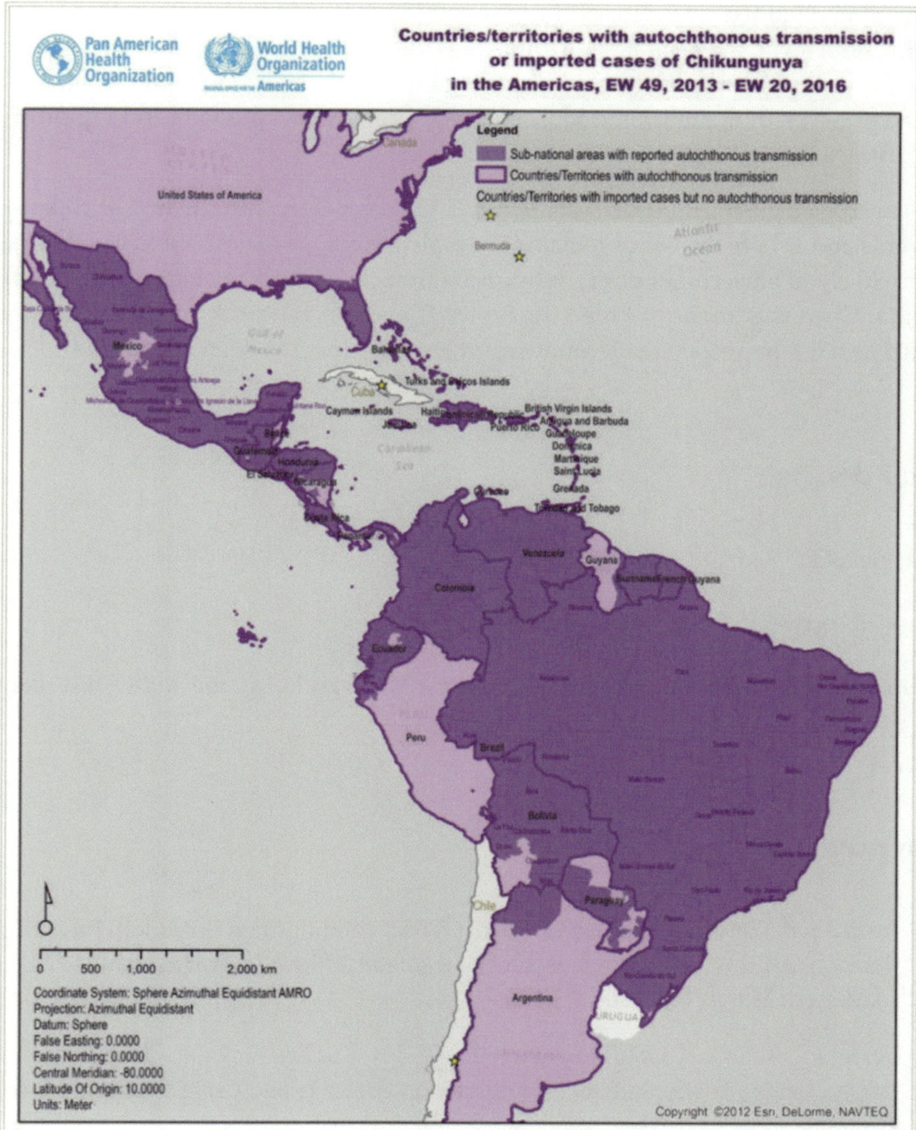

Figure 2. Countries/territories with autochthonous transmission or imported cases of chikungunya in the Americas, EW 49, 2013–EW 8, 2016.

a short time almost all the countries in the region are reporting indigenous cases with the exception of Chile and Uruguay (Figure 2).

Up to epidemiological week 8, in 2016, more than 1,800,000 cases across the continent have been reported since its introduction in 2013 [5].

In Chile chikungunya is still an infection to be expected in travelers to endemic areas, especially within Latin America and the Caribbean, which are the most frequent destination for Chilean tourists. Chikungunya is a disease to be considered in Chile for international travelers returning with fever and arthralgia. Arthralgia is the cardinal symptom and tends to be long-lasting. Preventive measures should be indicated to travelers visiting high-risk areas. As we have the presence of the mosquito in Continental Chile, autochthonous and imported cases will be expected.

Surveillance systems must be alert and sensible to detect early introduction of chikungunya to Easter Island, where the vector remains in a high percentage of households. In this scenario it is very likely to have chikungunya introduced from Tahiti as it has happened with dengue and Zika. Once chikungunya enters to Easter Island, an outbreak of great magnitude is expected as it has happened in all countries where this virus has been introduced.

Author details

Cecilia Perret P.*

Address all correspondence to: cperret@med.puc.cl

Pediatric Division, School of Medicine. Pontificia Universidad Católica de Chile. Santiago, Chile

References

[1] Instituto de Salud Pública de Chilehttp. Virus chikungunya [Internet]. July 2015 [Updated: 2015]. http://www.ispch.cl/sites/default/files/Chikungunya-21072015A.pdf [Accessed: March 10, 2016]

[2] Perret C., Abarca K.,Ovalle J., Ferrer P., Godoy P., Olea A., et al. Dengue-1 virus isolation during first dengue fever outbreak on Easter Island,Chile. Emerging Infectious Diseases. 2003;9(11):1465-1467.

[3] Cáceres C., Yung V., Araya P., Tognarelli J., Villagra E., Vera L., et al. Complete nucleotide sequence analysis of a Dengue-1 virus isolated on Easter Island, Chile. Archives of Virology. 2008;153(10):1967-1970.

[4] Tognarelli J., Ulloa S., Villagra E., Lagos J., Aguayo C., Fasce R. et al. A report on the outbreak of Zika virus on Easter Island, South Pacific, 2014. Archives of Virology. 2016;161(3):665-668. DOI: 10.1007/s00705-015-2695-5

[5] Panamerican Health Organization. Chikungunya: statistic data. Available on: http://www.paho.org/hq/index.php?option=com_topics&view=readall&cid=5927&Itemid=40931&lang=en [Accessed: March 11, 2016].

Chapter 4

The Eye and the Chikungunya Virus

Dayron Fernando Martínez-Pulgarín, Diana Marcela Muñoz-Urbano and Diego Zamora-de la Cruz

Additional information is available at the end of the chapter

http://dx.doi.org/10.5772/64474

Abstract

Ocular involvement in chikungunya virus (CHIKV) infection can be present as mild and vision-threatening ocular complications with unilateral or bilateral compromise in both gender and all ages. Precise prevalence and incidence are unknown, but ocular involvement of CHIKV infection is uncommon. Anterior uveitis is the most common syndromic manifestation; nevertheless the infection could manifest posterior segment repercussion, such as retinitis which is the other most usual clinical manifestation. At the beginning of the systemic disease, main ophthalmologic symptoms are conjunctival injection, retro-ocular pain, and photophobia. Ocular pathogenesis of CHIKV infection is not totally clarified; however, findings related to an immune dysregulation and proinflammatory processes are the most accepted theories. The diagnosis of CHIKV is based on polymerase chain reaction, virus isolation, or detection of viral antigens which should be used before the eighth day of systemic illness. After 8 days, chikungunya serologic tests such as IgM ELISA/rapid tests or IgG paired must be used. Actual management is focused according to the clinical context of each patient. While in most instances recovery of vision to normal occurs, CHIKV infection can result in blindness, the visual prognosis depends on various factors, but the common one is the early onset of corticosteroid treatment.

Keywords: Chikungunya virus, uveitis, retinitis, optic neuritis

1. Introduction

Ocular involvement in chikungunya virus (CHIKV) infection was unheard until the end of 2006 [1]. Since then, it has been demonstrated that CHIKV infection can cause both mild and vision-threatening ocular complications. Precise prevalence and incidence estimations of ocular manifestations in CHIKV infection are unknown, further have been reported to be uncommon [2–4].

In an attempt to determine the viral causes of anterior uveitis in a South Indian patient population, Babu et al. realized a retrospective nonrandomized study between January 2009 and July 2012; they found two cases of CHIKV-related anterior uveitis; among 36 patients included, the two of them had unilateral involvement [5].

The infection has plenty of ocular manifestations as reported in the case reports and case series; these could be present at the time of systemic illness or after resolution of systemic disease [1, 6, 7] but usually occurs after a latent period of a month to a year, but the presentation time also depends on the type of clinical presentation. Anterior uveitis and retinitis are the most common findings; with a typically benign clinical course, it has been reported that anterior uveitis affects more than 25% of the patients [2, 6, 8]. Posterior segment involvement may manifest as retinitis, choroiditis, neuroretinitis, and optic neuritis [1, 2, 7–11].

Commonly, in the acute phase of chikungunya fever, patients could manifest photophobia and retro-orbital pain [6, 12]; other ophthalmic manifestations of chikungunya virus infection include panuveitis, optic neuritis, keratitis, episcleritis, central retinal artery occlusion, exudative retinal detachment, lagophthalmos, and VIth nerve palsy [2, 6, 8, 13]; there are a variety of clinical manifestations that will be completely mentioned in other sections of this chapter.

Mittal et al. described a case series of 14 patients with confirmed CHIKV infection and optic neuritis; of them 42% had papillitis; 21% had retrobulbar neuritis; another 21% had optic tract involvement, and 16% had neuroretinitis [13]. Four years after this publication, Rose et al. reported an observational study involving 10 patients, who were confirmed cases of infection with CHIKV with acute optic neuritis. All 10 patients in the study presented with sudden onset decrease in vision and had a history of fever, joint pain, and skin rash. Among the 10 cases, 30% had bilateral disturbance and 70% had complaints only in one eye. The types of optic neuritis were unilateral papillitis (40%), bilateral papillitis (30%), retrobulbar neuritis (10%), perineuritis (10%), and neuroretinitis (10%) [10]. Meanwhile during 2011 a case of bilateral chikungunya neuroretinitis in a 65-year-old Asian-Indian, who presented with a month-old history of sudden, painless diminution of vision in both eyes and was treated with oral steroids and oral acyclovir for 3 weeks, was published, after which partial resolution was noted [14].

Meanwhile, Mahendradas et al. reported a different spectrum of ocular manifestations in nine patients with a positive serology for CHIKV: 55% had iridocyclitis, 33% had retinitis, and one patient of nine included had nodular episcleritis [8]. Conjunctivitis also been reported as a manifestation of CHIKV ocular infection, which looks like another viral infection and resolves spontaneously [9].

A report of the first known case of bilateral granulomatous panuveitis secondary to chikungunya fever in the United States, acquired by a US citizen traveling from an endemic region, was done by Scripsema et al.; they described a case of a 47-year-old woman presented with 10 days of bilateral decreased vision and photophobia with a concurrent febrile illness. Initially, she responded to corticosteroid treatment but developed recurrent inflammation 3 months after completing the initial treatment. Immunomodulatory therapy was initiated at the time of recurrence, and with this therapy alone, her inflammation has been controlled for 6 months.

http://dx.doi.org/10.5772/64474

In this article, the authors show that according to current reports of chikungunya fever-related uveitis with posterior inflammation, the distribution of presentation includes papillitis or optic neuritis (34%), neuroretinitis (12%), retrobulbar optic neuritis (14%), retinitis (11%), panuveitis (9%), choroiditis (7%), retrochiasmal or optic tract neuritis (7%), exudative retinal detachment (4%), and perineuritis (2%) [15].

Kalpana et al. presented a case series of 58 patients with Fuchs heterochromic iridocyclitis (FHI) and found one case caused by CHIKV; nevertheless the authors explain that it is difficult to speculate the association of FHI and chikungunya virus in this patient [16]. Before this case series, during 2010 Mahendradas et al. published the first report where the presence of chikungunya virus RNA has been associated with a case of bilateral Fuchs heterochromic iridocyclitis, although the authors clear that it is not accurate if the chikungunya virus was the initiator of the disease or a coincidental finding [17].

Ocular involvement caused by chikungunya virus should be included in the differential diagnosis, especially in the endemic areas, of any patient presenting with ocular manifestations and a history of fever, even more when this is accompanied by suggestive symptoms of an infection caused by CHIKV [18]. This chapter describes the most important aspects of the ocular compromise caused by CHIKV, items that the clinicians should consider when approaching a patient with a suspected ocular involvement by the mentioned virus.

2. Ocular pathogenesis

Ophthalmologic involvement due to chikungunya virus infection is a state that affects plenty of structures of the eyeball including the eyelids, conjunctiva, cornea, sclera, episclera, iris, retina, optic nerve, etc. This diversity of ocular findings has been mainly associated with the most recent outbreaks of the virus because of genomic variations resulting in different virus strains with changes in activity and virulence. The outbreak of the disease in La Réunion, an island in Indian Ocean, is related to a different strain of the virus which has been associated with a higher replication rate than West African and Asian strains of chikungunya virus according to studies in animals [19, 20]. It is not pretty clear the exact pathogenic mechanism through chikungunya virus makes its disturbances in different tissues, especially the eye; however a group of successive steps has been proposed to describe the cycle of infection that applies for systemic and ocular disease (Figure 1) [19, 21].

The initial response of the body involves an elevation of type I interferon levels and a hypersensitivity reaction mediated by antibodies against viral antigens causing joint symptoms and the possible beginning of ocular compromise [21]. The existence of a huge controversy about the determination of target cells compromised by chikungunya virus has marked the research pattern in the last years in an attempt to create new therapeutic interventions. Some researches in recent years have determined that fibroblasts, endothelium and epithelium cells, and macrophages are susceptible to infection by chikungunya virus, especially by La Réunion strain, leading to apoptosis in some cases [22]. Different studies made in mice and humans have found that fibroblasts are the major cell target for chikungunya virus, including those in

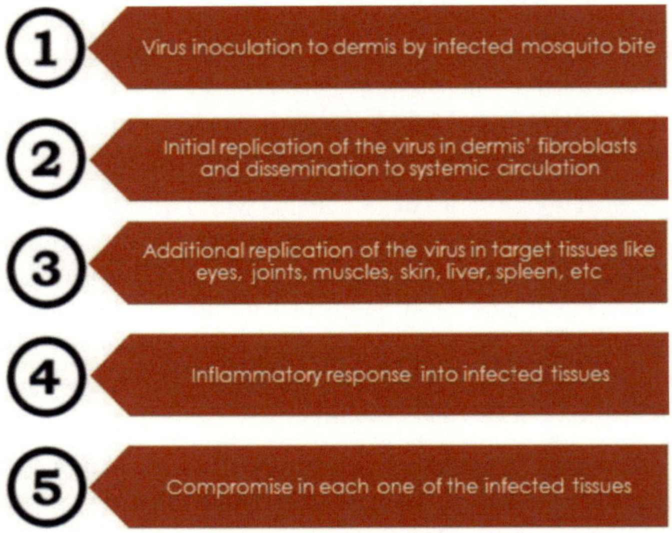

Figure 1. Systemic and ocular pathogenic process of chikungunya virus infection. Based on Couderc T and Lecuit M. Chikungunya virus pathogenesis: From bedside to bench. Antiviral Res. 2015;121:120-131.

eyeball tissues, something that can be explained by their reticular network formed by gap junctions making possible dissemination from cell to cell; nevertheless the exact mechanism has not been described [23, 24].

In the eye, the cornea commitment depends on the infection of epithelial and endothelial cells, which are the target cells of chikungunya virus at this level. There is evidence about the potential risk of transmission of chikungunya virus through corneal graft transplantation. According to Courdec et al., they identified a group of corneal donors who were seropositive for CHIKV IgM and/or IgG, and their samples showed evidence of the presence of the virus after the conventional eye bank preservation methods, which were ineffective to inactivate the virus from the corneal samples, and conclude that CHIKV can be transmitted via ocular route in humans, coinciding with studies made in immunocompetent mice demonstrating that the corneal tissue infected with chikungunya virus in replication state that was inoculated onto scarified cornea leads to viral transmission in the studied mice [24]. This study also determined that the presence of replication-competent virus in the eye did not correlate with viral detection in the blood or the presence of antiviral antibodies. Other sites in the eyeball like the scleral connective tissue, stroma of smooth muscles of ciliary bodies, and stroma of the iris, the fibroblast is the ideal cell for the virus because of its high rate of replication that leads to a huge production of infectious viral particles. Besides, there have also been signals of infection between fibers of ocular muscles [25].

Involvement of the optic nerve is not pretty clear; nevertheless it is presumed that an immune dysregulation, superantigen induction, hypersensitivity reaction, and molecular mimicry between stimulating virus-derived antigens and normal or altered host tissue proteins may be the causes of the optic nerve damage [10, 13, 26, 27].

There are descriptions about fluctuations in the values of intraocular pressure when inflammatory processes in anterior segment occur. Hypotension may occur when a loss of integrity of the blood-aqueous barrier exists leading to an increased aqueous humor flow. Episodes of ocular hypertension happen when inflammation of trabecular system appears, leading to obstruction of aqueous humor flow [28].

There is a theory that serves as a complement for chikungunya pathogenesis, including the ocular compromise, and consists of an increased production of chemokines, like interleukin-8 (IL-8) and monocyte chemoattractant protein 1(MCP1), by infected monocyte-derived macrophages. However, this last theory is just a hypothesis based on studies made using the Ross River virus, which is a virus that belongs to alphavirus family, as the chikungunya virus; therefore it can keep some behavior similarities with CHIKV [23, 29]. Primary cultures of B and T cells, monocytes, and monocyte-derived dendritic cells were found not to be susceptible to CHIKV infection in vitro [19, 22, 30].

In summary, ocular pathogenesis in context of CHIKV infection is a process that is not totally clarified, despite the progressively increase in research about this field in recent years; however, findings related to an immune dysregulation state and proinflammatory processes are the most accepted theories and could guide the course of ophthalmologic research about this field in the coming years.

3. Clinical findings

Ophthalmologic manifestations due to chikungunya infection are a set of pathologies that cause different degrees of damages, involving plenty of structures on anterior and posterior pole during the course of the systemic disease, even after its resolution with a latent period of a month to a year [6, 31], and can be present as both mild and vision-threatening ocular complications with unilateral or bilateral compromise in both gender and all ages [32], being retinitis and uveitis the most common syndromic manifestations. At the beginning of the systemic disease, main visible clinical symptoms are conjunctival injection, retro-ocular pain, and photophobia [2, 12, 33]; meanwhile other existing symptoms like blurred vision, floaters, epiphora, irritation, and diplopia usually appear after a latent period of a month to a year (during chronic phase) [16, 32, 34].

The time between beginning of fever and the onset of ophthalmologic symptoms is unknown; however some retrospective researches in an attempt to determine this interval have shown that involvement of visual acuity initiates approximately 4 weeks after fever begins, pain and floaters can be present after 12 weeks, and redness can appear 10–12 weeks after fever onset [8]; nevertheless these intervals can fluctuate according to the specific affected ocular structure and the degree of involvement. Also, the small number of patients used by researchers in these studies makes accurate data on these aspects too difficult to reach, but initial approximations like this allow the creation of bigger studies that make possible to find high-impact data.

Ocular manifestations of chikungunya virus can keep some similarities with other viruses like dengue and Zika. Dengue ocular manifestations are uncommon but can be present particularly in young adults with a mean age of early 30s and without any sex predilection, debuting when platelets are at lowest count, especially one week after fever onset [18].The most common ocular findings due to dengue fever are subconjunctival hemorrhage, dengue maculopathy, anterior uveitis, vitreitis, retinal pigment epithelium mottling, foveolitis, retinochoroiditis, choroidal effusion, optic disk swelling, optic neuritis, neuroretinitis, panophthalmitis, retinal hemorrhages, and oculomotor nerve palsy [31, 32, 34].

Zika ocular manifestations are included in the category of "atypical"; however the ophthalmologic manifestations which have been described in literature until now are the non-mucopurulent conjunctivitis and the retro-ocular pain. In a Yap island population when an outbreak of Zika virus was informed, about 55% of cases were reported with the presence of non-mucopurulent conjunctivitis and 39% of cases with retro-ocular pain; uveitis and different ocular inflammatory processes were not reported [35]. Differential diagnosis with dengue and chikungunya viruses should be based in all manifestations and not purely based on ophthalmologic findings [36].

3.1. Anterior uveitis

Anterior uveitis, including granulomatous and non-granulomatous variety, is the main ocular condition due to infection caused by chikungunya virus [2]. There is no evidence that demonstrates that uveitis secondary to chikungunya virus has a different behavior than uveitis caused by other etiologies, particularly those from other arboviruses such as dengue [37]. It is defined as an inflammation of the uveal tract, specifically the iris and pars plicata of the ciliary body. The presence of symptoms can be insidious or sudden, taking between a few weeks to a few months to resolve. Main clinical manifestations include pain, photophobia, conjunctival injection, hypopyon (the presence of inflammatory cells in anterior chamber and according to their number represents ocular disease activity), epiphora, and pigmented central globular keratic precipitates with an infiltrative and dendritic pattern on the surface of the corneal endothelium in some cases (Figure 2.) [38].

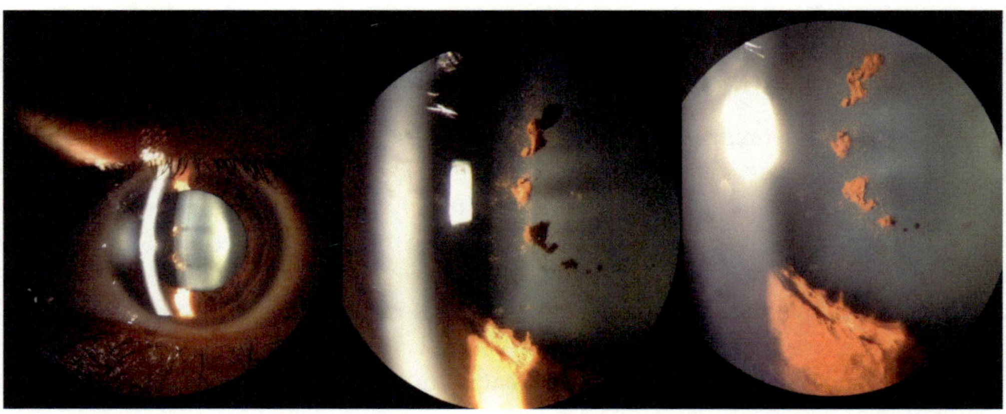

Figure 2. Pigmented keratic precipitates at cornea. Picture took by Diego Zamora-de la Cruz.

http://dx.doi.org/10.5772/64474

The visual acuity can be affected depending on severity and activity state of the uveitis; miosis can be present, making a predisposition to formation of posterior synechia, which is the main complication related to anterior uveitis [12, 39]. Funduscopy is usually normal, but it should always be realized for excluding anterior uveitis due to an infection by toxoplasma or acute retinal necrosis in posterior pole. It is possible to develop high intraocular pressure in the context of an open corneoscleral angle [32]. It is clearly established that chikungunya anterior uveitis can imitate a herpetic anterior variety [40]. However, we can differentiate both: In the first one the compromise is more bilateral [41], exists past history of fever with joint pain, have being in endemic areas [33, 42, 43], and there are positive serologic results [12, 32, 41].

Ocular compromise by CHIKV could manifest also as Fuchs heterochromic iridocyclitis (FHI), which is a disease of unknown etiology characterized by low-grade intraocular inflammation, iris heterochromia and/or atrophy, keratic precipitates with stellate morphology with fibrillary extensions, the absence of synechiae, development of cataract, and in few cases increased intraocular pressure; however this syndrome has been much more linked to other infections and noninfectious diseases than chikungunya virus (Figure 3.) [16].

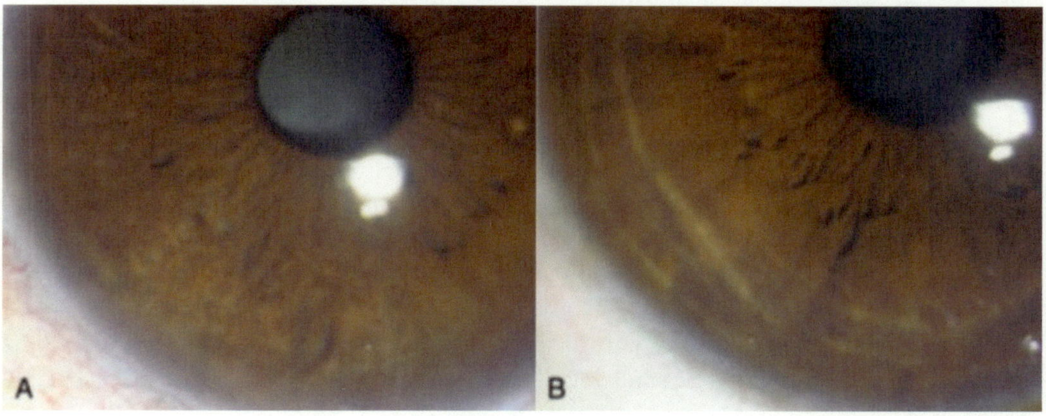

Figure 3. Fuchs heterochromic iridocyclitis: (A) normal eye and (B) affected eye. Taken from Babu K, Adiga M, Govekar S, Kumar B, and Murthy K. Associations of Fuchs heterochromic iridocyclitis in a South Indian patient population. *Journal of Ophthalmic Inflammation and Infection*. 2013; 3(14). Reproduced with permission.

According to case reports, a past history of systemic symptoms of chikungunya was reported in the previous 1–6 weeks; the affectation by FHI was more unilateral with a mean age of 37.95 ± 12.42 years (range from 16 to 68 years), and the most common complaint of patients is blurred vision. Despite these results, it still remains unclear the exact time of the presence of viral antigen in the aqueous, so it can be difficult to assume a causal role of chikungunya virus in FHI cases [16, 17, 44].

3.2. Posterior uveitis

Posterior uveitis is less common than anterior uveitis in the context of infection by chikungunya virus, and it is defined as inflammation of the choroid and/or retina, vitreous, optic nerve head, and retinal vessels. According to the Standardization of Uveitis Nomenclature (SUN) working group, posterior uveitis includes focal, multifocal, or diffuse choroiditis, chorioretinitis, retinochoroiditis, retinitis, neuroretinitis, and retinal vasculitis [39, 45, 46]. Clinical signs might be varied according to the structure involved. Decreased vision, central scotoma, peripheral field defects, and color vision defect can be present. Symptoms in the anterior segment like conjunctival injection, pain, and hypopyon are less frequent [32].

3.2.1. Retinitis

Retinitis onset occurs between 2 and 4 weeks after febrile period of systemic disease. According to some authors, this interval can support the hypothesis that ocular lesions could be an immune-mediated process rather than a direct viral effect [47]. It can be focal, multifocal, or diffuse. Patients consult with a history of sudden vision lost without pain. Active lesions are characterized by retinal whitish opacities, poorly demarcated by surrounding edema [39]. It is usually accompanied by mild vitreitis, retinal hemorrhages, compromise of retinal vessels, and the presence of areas of retinal whitening in the posterior pole [48]. Funduscopy allows visualizing focal and multifocal patches of retinitis macular edema, serous detachment at the macula, and localized involvement of the retinal vessel [49]. It is described that retinitis caused by chikungunya fever can simulate herpetic and West Nile virus retinitis; thus the importance of anamnesis lies in the identification of systemic symptoms of chikungunya infection, making possible the differentiation to other etiologies [50, 51].

3.2.2. Choroiditis

Choroiditis can be, as retinitis, focal, multifocal, or diffuse. It usually does not produce vitreitis in the absence of concomitant retinal involvement. Choroiditis active lesion is characterized by a round yellow nodule in any part of the choroid tissue, especially the iris. Vasculitis includes a compromise of arteries and veins (periarteritis and periphlebitis), and it is characterized by a perivascular irregular yellow or white cuff and can be associated with hemorrhages [39].

3.3. Optic neuritis

Optic neuritis is an inflammatory, infectious, or demyelinating process that involves optic nerve. According to funduscopy, it can be classified as retrobulbar neuritis, papillitis, or neuroretinitis. There exists another classification based on etiology, which is divided into demyelinating, parainfectious, infectious, and noninfectious optic neuritis. In the case of optic neuritis due to chikungunya infection, it belongs to parainfectious class, which occurs after the viral infection [39]. Optic neuritis is characterized by acute or subacute loss of vision, pain with ocular movements, and color vision defects. Papillitis is the most often clinical sign according to observational case series. Patients report the presence of blurred vision after a mean of 11.0±14.0 days of a symptom-free period, and the ocular symptoms had a mean duration of 14 days [10, 13].

3.4. Corneal involvement

Keratitis and keratouveitis are the main conditions that affect corneal tissue in the context of chikungunya infection. It is an inflammatory process of the cornea. There is no defined time between systemic symptoms and the onset of corneal compromise; however there are some studies which affirm that viral infection at the corneal cell can remain asymptomatic for some periods of time, approximately 1 month according to case reports [3, 25]. Blurred vision and ocular irritation are some of the associated symptoms, and involvement of corneal surface can include bilateral punctate superficial keratitis and stromal immune ring formation with underlying keratic precipitates which can resolve after 2 weeks of topical corticoid therapy (Figure 2) [2, 3].

3.5. Episcleritis

Episcleritis is defined as inflammation of the episclera, which is the most external layer of sclera. It is classified as simple or nodular. Regardless of the cause of the pathology, it has a pattern to recur in the same eye in posterior episodes [39]. Simple episcleritis is characterized by localized conjunctival injection with a duration of 12 hours approximately. Nodular episcleritis is represented by conjunctival injection that becomes bigger progressively with the presence of painful nodules localized almost all the time at the interpalpebral fissure. Episcleritis has a benign and self-limited course with a total conservation of vision and an excellent prognosis [8].

3.6. Panophthalmitis

Panophthalmitis in seropositive chikungunya patients is an unusual manifestation by this agent. It is characterized by an inflammatory process of all structures in the eye. The only case report on the literature of this manifestation related to chikungunya was in a middle-aged male patient who presented with painful progressive proptosis with loss of vision in the left eye over a period of 6 hours with a history of fever, rash, and severe joint pain in the previous five days. Moreover, the patient presented at physical examination visual acuity with no light perception, swelling, and redness of both eyelids, raised temperature over the lids, and proptosis. Despite panophthalmitis is a very rare manifestation, its rapid fulminating course and severity of symptoms make this one of the most feared ocular manifestations [52].

4. Ophthalmologic diagnosis

As discussed in the additional chapters, the diagnosis of CHIKV is based on polymerase chain reaction, virus isolation, or detection of viral antigens which should be used before the eighth day of systemic illness. After 8 days, chikungunya serologic tests such as IgM ELISA/rapid tests or IgG paired must be used because the viral load will have decreased [53].

Actually, it has not been possible to find any standard method for ocular CHIKV infection; however according to some authors, the collection of aqueous humor can be useful for the determination of virus [12, 17], as it was previously documented in a patient who underwent cataract surgery [17]. Despite this report, it is not recommended to take samples of aqueous or vitreous humor if the illness does not threat the integrity or eye function because of the possibility to cause a superimposed infection.

Collection of aqueous humor can be made through puncture that is performed before phacoemulsification surgery or by taking aqueous samples in the lens remains collection bag and supplemented with the implementation of reverse transcription polymerase chain reaction (RT-PCR) [12, 17].

Mahendradas et al. demonstrated that only the aqueous or vitreous humor and no other tissues such as the anterior lens capsule can become infected by the virus [17]. It is important to recognize clinically if the inflammation is related to the virus and latent preconditions as some other viral infections or systemic diseases that trigger the clinical manifestation.

Other tests could be used such as ELISA, immunochromatographic test, hemagglutination inhibition, or neutralization techniques, which allow diagnosing indirectly the virus infection through quantification of the IgM and IgG antibodies in serum; however, these are too much unspecific [12].

To date, the RT-PCR is considered as the gold standard test to identify the etiologic agent in ocular tissue involvement because of its high specificity and sensitivity rates. The RT-PCR must be taken when viremia is active (109–1012 viral copies per ml of blood) [52].

As reported by some authors [12, 17], cataract postoperative state of patients with chikungunya is similar to patients with chronic uveitis; therefore, it must be considered to continue topical and systemic steroids in the postoperative period.

The definitive diagnosis has to be made by integrating systemic clinical findings with serologic test for CHIKV. The differential diagnosis is usually made with anterior/posterior uveitis caused by herpes simplex virus (HSV) and retinitis due to West Nile virus [12].

The panophthalmitis is a global inflammatory process of the eyeball due to CHIKV which has been reported in the literature [52], but the association between chikungunya and panophthalmitis is doubtful and requires further investigation; according to Rajan and colleagues, no evidence of viral agent was found in the ocular tissue.

It is relevant to say that ocular diagnosis of CHIKV has to be always considered as an exclusion diagnosis, after probing more common etiologies of clinical manifestation mentioned above.

Fluoroangiography and spectral domain optical coherence tomography (SD-OCT) are additional tests that can be used for ocular chikungunya infection. The first one can reveal unspecific findings of neuroretinitis, macular edema, and even serous retinal detachments associated with chikungunya. The use of these tests is not recommended for diagnosis but to check evolution of inflammatory process. For instance, in retinitis cases analyzed with fluoroangiography, hypofluorescent areas in late stages of the study are observed; meanwhile SD-OCT revealed increased reflectivity in the nerve fiber layer zone which can be associated with serous retinal detachments (Figure 4). Nevertheless, it is so relevant to remind that the main goal of these studies is to follow up the patient's clinical course of the ocular disease [8, 12].

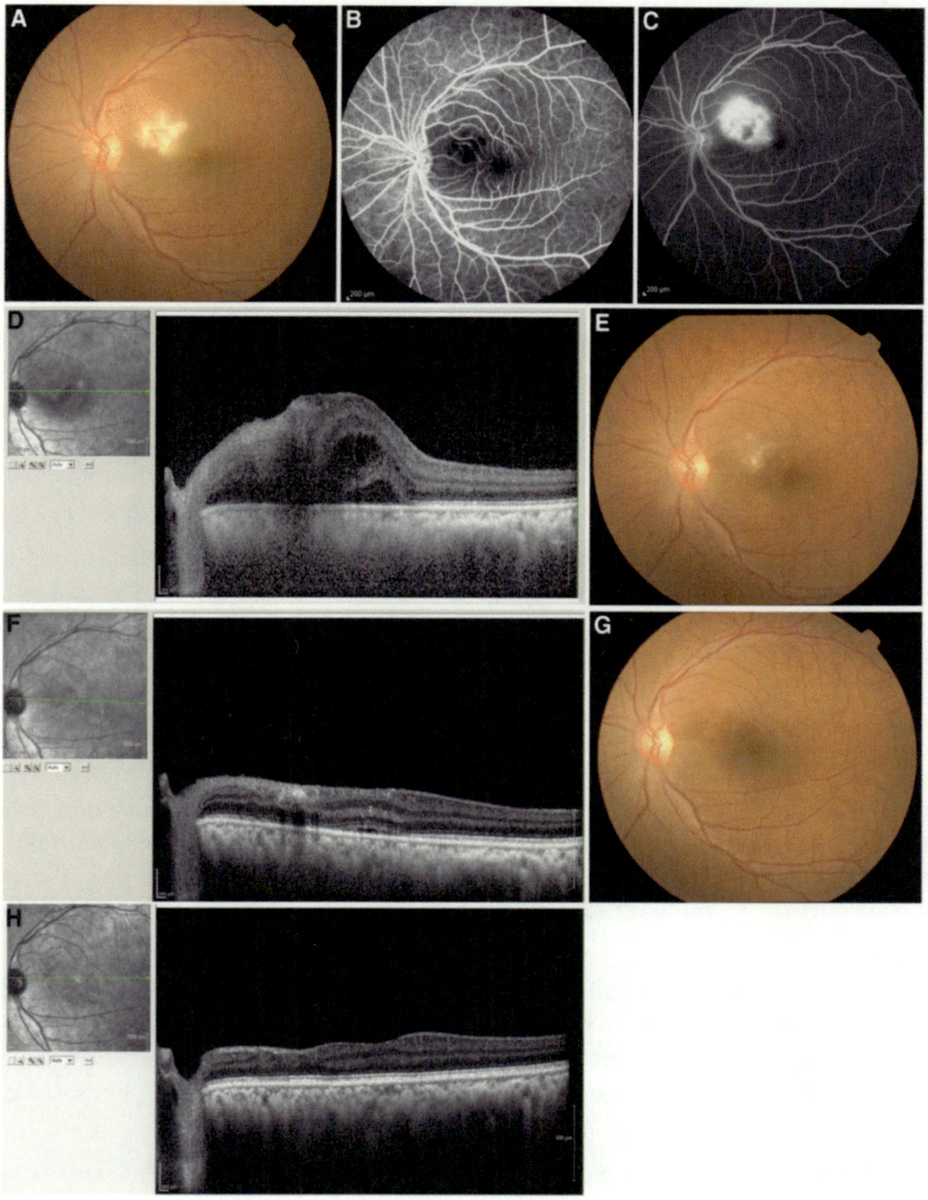

Figure 4. Retinitis findings in SD-OCT and fluoroangiography. (A) Fundus photograph of the left eye showing confluent area of retinal whitening suggestive of retinitis. (B) Fundus fluorescein angiography with early hypofluorescence in the posterior pole, and (C) late hyperfluorescence in the posterior pole. (D) Spectral domain optical coherence tomography (SD-OCT) revealed an increased reflectivity in the nerve fiber layer zone corresponding to the areas of retinitis with after shadowing and fluid-filled spaces in the outer retina with serous retinal detachment. (E) Fundus photograph showing resolving retinitis lesion 2 weeks after initiation of systemic steroid therapy. (F) SD-OCT showing decreased area of hyperreflectivity in the inner retina with resolving retinal detachment. (G) Fundus photograph after 4 months, showing complete resolution of retinitis. (H) SD-OCT showing resolution of retinitis with thinning of the inner retinal layers nasal to the fovea. Taken from Mahendradas P, Avadhani K, Shetty R. Chikungunya and the eye: a review. *Journal of Ophthalmic Inflammation and Infection*. 2013; 3(35). Reproduced with permission.

5. Treatment

There is no specific antiviral treatment for the CHIKV ocular infection to date. Actual treatment for ocular manifestations due to this virus is focused on control of symptoms and avoidance of complications resulting from inflammation of ocular tissues [12].

Systemically, the treatment is based on handling inflammation with corticosteroids and immunomodulators. The treatment is focused according to the clinical context of each patient. In a patient with an active viral process and an inflammatory ocular event, other causes of retinitis, scleritis, and uveitis must be excluded.

Murthy et al. reported a case of bilateral retinitis due to a systemic infection of CHIKV. Inflammation secondary to HSV was documented, and the treatment was made with intravenous and oral acyclovir, intravitreal ganciclovir, and oral corticoids and focused on decreasing the viral copies. The role of acyclovir in treatment against ocular CHIKV should be restricted to cases where CHIKV and HSV concomitant infection is present or when an inefficient response to anti-inflammatory therapy exists; however, this is still a controversial fact [46, 47].

As soon as ocular inflammation appears, it is convenient to assess the systemic condition of the patient, with the purpose of identifying contraindications for systemic steroids use, with the objectives to reduce eye inflammation and prevent irreversible blindness. Nowadays, treatment is focused only on treating uveitis complications due to CHIKV [8, 12, 38].

5.1. Local treatment

In all patients who experience active anterior segment inflammation, it is preferred to start treatment with prednisolone acetate 0.2%, eight times a day, with a reductive dose schedule every 5 days depending on patient response. It is preferred to add cyclopentolate 1.0% twice a day or tropicamide with phenylephrine every 8 hours, allowing not only the patient cycloplegia but also iris mobilization, avoiding the formation of posterior synechiae [41].

Occasionally, patients may experience increased intraocular pressure in the context of uveitis, which can be controlled by adding a topical treatment with timolol 0.5% twice daily. It is relevant to remind the mechanism by which the increase of intraocular pressure occurs. High levels of prostaglandins can increase production of aqueous humor, and the presence of trabeculitis leads to an obstruction of the aqueous humor flow, increasing intraocular pressure [41].

It is recommended to use some topical nonsteroidal anti-inflammatory drugs to create synergy with steroid and reduce rapidly the present symptoms. Some examples can include nepafenac every 12 hours, bromfenac every 6 hours, or topical ketorolac every 8 hours [41].

5.2. Systemic treatment

Once any contraindication to initiate steroids is excluded, intravenous steroids may be started if inflammatory events such as optical neuritis or any other threatening visual condition are documented. In the cases of increased refractory intraocular pressure to topical treatment, it is recommended to add acetazolamide 250 mg twice daily for three days, taking care of the renal function [41].

6. Visual prognosis

While in most instances recovery of vision to normal occurs, CHIKV infection can result in blindness; especially if it courses in association with optic neuritis or neuroretinitis, patients may present sudden loss of vision caused by chikungunya fever associated with optic neuritis [4, 10, 18]; this manifestation of the ocular infection may have a progressive visual loss and may occur rapidly over several hours or over days [10]. Some authors suggest that visual prognosis is good with anterior segment involvement, whereas that with posterior segment involvement (retinochoroiditis) is poor [2, 18, 32, 54], though later certain aspects that greatly influence the visual forecast will be mentioned.

The majority of patients with retinitis have a good visual outcome over a 10- to 12-week period [12]. It has been described that alterations like granulomatous and non-granulomatous uveitis, optic neuritis, and dendritic lesions are common lesions with good visual prognosis, but as noted above, the prognosis is influenced by several aspects, and this is dependent of each clinical context [2]. On the other hand, macular ischemia and optic disk changes account for the poor visual outcome seen in a minority of patients [12, 55].

Unlike previously exposed, Mahesh G et al. reported a case of a 48-year-old female with bilateral neuroretinitis; the patient received early systemic steroids since she had optic disk involvement, and visual recovery was very satisfactory [1]. Rapid visual recovery is usually the norm with immediate administration of systemic steroid therapy [10, 13]. An observational case series that included 14 patients with clinical features of CHIKV infection and associated optic neuritis reported complete or partial improvement of vision in 71% of patients with good response to steroids if given early in the course of illness; in this study, the researchers presented three patients in whom treatment was initiated 1 month after the onset of visual symptoms for whom there was no visual improvement [13].

Nonce, Chanana et al. [7] reported a case of a 16-year-old male patient with bilateral macular choroiditis following chikungunya virus infection that started treatment with oral prednisolone; he showed evidence of resolving choroiditis bilaterally within 6 weeks of treatment, but the vision did not improve further [7].

In an observational study involving 10 patients, whose cases of infection with CHIKV with acute optic neuritis were confirmed, the overall prognosis in terms of visual acuity, color vision, pupillary reaction, and visual field was favorable. They received intravenous methylprednisolone for 3 days, followed by oral prednisolone in a tapering dose; the authors emphasize the importance of prompt establishment of corticosteroid therapy to lead to rapid recovery of visual function in patients with acute presentation of optic neuritis, but it has no role when treatment is initiated at a late stage of the disease [10].

A retrospective study showed 14 consecutive cases who presented to the Vitreo Retina Department of the Minto Ophthalmic Hospital; of them one patient was positive for IgM chikungunya; she had bilateral anterior non-granulomatous uveitis and retinitis with optic nerve involvement in one eye; the patient showed a favorable response to oral prednisolone; the dose was tapered based on clinical response over a period of 6 weeks improving from an average of 2/60 to 6/24 vision [49]. In a similar way, a case series that included nine chikungunya patients with ocular involvement found a benign course in the cases of iridocyclitis and episcleritis; they showed complete resolution, with preservation of vision, and patients that presented with retinitis showed gradual resolution over a period of 6 to 8 weeks with systemic acyclovir and the corticosteroids [8].

Other less fortunate cases have been reported, in which there is no any treatment that can improve final visual prognosis, such as one of the patients with acute necrotizing panophthalmitis; although the CHIKV was not isolated from vitreous tap, chorioretinal biopsy, and other eviscerated materials, the serological studies were positive with high titer of recent infection. The case resulted in a painful blind eye, which required evisceration [52].

During April of 2015, Hayek et al. reported the first case of a teen girl with CHIKV-induced stromal keratouveitis; she had complete resolution of the corneal infiltrate after 2 weeks of topical corticosteroid treatment [3]. As previously described, the visual prognosis depends on various factors, but the common one that is found in the scientific literature is the early onset of corticosteroid treatment. However there is no specific agent that was found effective against the chikungunya virus. Most of the infected patients with CHIKV are treated symptomatically, and it is not completely clear whether any therapy is effective in improving the visual prognosis [8].

Author details

Dayron Fernando Martínez-Pulgarín[1*], Diana Marcela Muñoz-Urbano[1] and Diego Zamora-de la Cruz[2]

*Address all correspondence to: dayronfernando@hotmail.com

1 Research Group and Incubator Public Health and Infection, Faculty of Health Sciences, Universidad Tecnológica de Pereira, Pereira, Risaralda, Colombia

2 Institute of Ophthalmology, Conde de Valenciana Foundation, México City, México

References

[1] Mahesh G., Giridhar A., Shedbele A., Kumar R., Saikumar S.J. A case of bilateral presumed chikungunya neuroretinitis. Indian Journal of Ophthalmology. 2009;57(2): 148-150. DOI: 10.4103/0301-4738.45508.

[2] Lalitha P., Rathinam S., Banushree K., Maheshkumar S., Vijayakumar R., Sathe P. Ocular involvement associated with an epidemic outbreak of chikungunya virus infection. American Journal of Ophthalmology. 2007;144(4):552-556. DOI: 10.1016/j.ajo. 2007.06.002.

[3] Hayek S., Rousseau A., Bouthry E., Prat C.M., Labetoulle M. Chikungunya virus infection and bilateral stromal keratouveitis. JAMA Ophthalmology. 2015;133(7): 849-850. DOI: 10.1001/jamaophthalmol.2015.0698.

[4] Rajapakse S., Rodrigo C., Rajapakse A. Atypical manifestations of chikungunya infection. Transactions of the Royal Society of Tropical Medicine and Hygiene. 2010;104(2):89-96. DOI: 10.1016/j.trstmh.2009.07.031.

[5] Babu K., Kini R., Philips M., Subbakrishna D.K. Clinical profile of isolated viral anterior uveitis in a South Indian patient population. Ocular Immunology & Inflammation. 2014;22(5):356-359. DOI: 10.3109/09273948.2013.841482.

[6] Khairallah M., Yahia S.B., Attia S. Arthropod vector-borne uveitis in the developing world. International Ophthalmology Clinics. 2010;50(2):125-144.

[7] Chanana B., Azad R.V., Nair S. Bilateral macular choroiditis following chikungunya virus infection. Eye (Lond). 2007;21(7):1020-1021. DOI: 10.1038/sj.eye.6702862.

[8] Mahendradas P., Ranganna S.K., Shetty R., Balu R., Narayana K.M., Babu R.B., et al. Ocular manifestations associated with chikungunya. Ophthalmology. 2008;115(2): 287-291. DOI: 10.1016/j.ophtha.2007.03.085.

[9] Parola P., de Lamballerie X., Jourdan J., Rovery C., Vaillant V., Minodier P., et al. Novel chikungunya virus variant in travelers returning from Indian ocean islands. Emerging Infectious Diseases. 2006;12(10):1493-1499.

[10] Rose N., Anoop T.M., John A.P., Jabbar P.K., George K.C. Acute optic neuritis following infection with chikungunya virus in southern rural India. International Journal of Infectious Diseases. 2011;15(2):e147-150. DOI: 10.1016/j.ijid.2010.10.004.

[11] Dunn J.P. Uveitis. Primary Care: Clinics in Office Practice. 2015;42(3):305-323. DOI: 10.1016/j.pop.2015.05.003.

[12] Mahendradas P., Avadhani K., Shetty R. Chikungunya and the eye: a review. Journal of Ophthalmic Inflammation and Infection. 2013;3(35):1-9.

[13] Mittal A., Mittal S., Bharati M.J., Ramakrishnan R., Saravanan S., Sathe P.S. Optic neuritis associated with chikungunya virus infection in south India. Archives of Ophthalmology. 2007;125(10):1381-1386.

[14] Nair A.G., Biswas J., Bhende M.P. A case of bilateral chikungunya neuroretinitis. Journal of Ophthalmic Inflammation and Infection. 2012;2(1):39-40. DOI: 10.1007/s12348-011-0038-6.

[15] Scripsema N.K., Sharif E., Samson C.M., Kedhar S., Rosen R.B. Chikungunya—associated uveitis and exudative retinal detachment: a case report. Retinal Cases & Brief Reports. 2015;9:352-356.

[16] Babu K., Adiga M., Govekar S.R., Kumar B.V., Murthy K.R. Associations of Fuchs heterochromic iridocyclitis in a south Indian patient population. Journal of Opthalmic Inflammation and Infection. 2013;3(14). DOI: 10.1186/1869-5760-3-14.

[17] Mahendradas P., Shetty R., Malathi J., Madhavan H.N. Chikungunya virus iridocyclitis in Fuchs' heterochromic iridocyclitis. Indian Journal of Ophthalmology. 2010;58(6):545-547. DOI: 10.4103/0301-4738.71707.

[18] Ranjan R., Ranjan S. Ocular pathology: role of emerging viruses in the asia-pacific region-a review. Asia Pacific Journal of Ophthalmology. 2014;3(5):299-307. DOI: 10.1097/APO.0000000000000021.

[19] Couderc T., Lecuit M. Chikungunya virus pathogenesis: from bedside to bench. Antiviral Research. 2015;121:120-131. DOI: 10.1016/j.antiviral.2015.07.002.

[20] Messaoudi I., Vomaske J., Totonchy T., Kreklywich C.N., Haberthur K., Springgay L., et al. Chikungunya virus infection results in higher and persistent viral replication in aged rhesus macaques due to defects in anti-viral immunity. PLoS Neglected Tropical Diseases. 2013;7(7). DOI: 10.1371/journal.pntd.0002343.

[21] Weaver S.C., Lecuit M. Chikungunya virus and the global spread of a mosquito-borne disease. The New England Journal of Medicine. 2015;372(13):1231-1239. DOI: 10.1056/NEJMra1406035.

[22] Sourisseau M., Schilte C., Casartelli N., Trouillet C., Guivel-Benhassine F., Rudnicka D.,et al. Characterization of reemerging chikungunya virus. PLoS Pathogens. 2007;3(6):804-817.

[23] Pardigon, N. The biology of chikungunya: a brief review of what we still do not know. Pathologie Biologie. 2009;57(2):127-132. DOI: 10.1016/j.patbio.2008.02.016.

[24] Couderc T., Chretien F., Schilte C., Disson O., Brigitte M., Guivel-Benhassine F., et al. A mouse model for Chikungunya: young age and inefficient type-I interferon signaling are risk factors for severe disease. PLoS Pathogens. 2008;4(2). DOI: 10.1371/journal.ppat.0040029.

[25] Couderc T., Gangneux N., Chretien F., Caro V., Le Luong T., Ducloux B., et al. Chikungunya virus infection of corneal grafts. The Journal of Infectious Diseases. 2012;206(6):851-859. DOI: 10.1093/infdis/jis296.

[26] Schuffenecker I., Iteman I., Michault A., Murri S., Frangeul L., Vaney M.C., et al. Genome microevolution of chikungunya viruses causing the Indian Ocean outbreak. PLoS Medicine. 2006;3(7):1058-1070. DOI: 10.1371/journal.pmed.0030263.

[27] Thorne J.E., Jabs D.A. The eye in rheumatic disease. Duane's Ophthalmology.2013 ed. Lippincott Williams & Wilkin. Philadelphia. 2013. pp. 297-303.

[28] Bodh S.A., Kumar V., Raina U.K., Ghosh B., Thakar M. Inflammatory glaucoma. Oman Journal of Ophthalmology. 2011;4(1):3-9. DOI: 10.4103/0974-620X.77655.

[29] Luis Mateo L., Linn M.L., McColl S.R., Cross S., Gardner J., Suhrbier A. An arthrogenic alphavirus induces monocyte chemoattractant protein-1 and interleukin-8. Intervirology. 2000;43:55-60.

[30] Teng T.S., Foo S.S., Simamarta D., Lum F.M., Teo T.H., Lulla A., et al.. Viperin restricts chikungunya virus replication and pathology. The Journal of Clinical Investigation. 2012;122(12):4447-4460. DOI: 10.1172/JCI63120.

[31] Khairallah M., Jelliti B., Attia S. Uveitis in the developing world. Expert Review of Ophthalmology. 2010;5(2):161-176.

[32] Khairallah M., Chee S.P., Rathinam S.R., Attia S., Nadella V. Novel infectious agents causing uveitis. International Ophthalmology. 2010;30(5):465-483. DOI: 10.1007/s10792-009-9319-6.

[33] Center for Disease Control and Prevention. Chikungunya fever diagnosed among international travelers. Morbidity and Mortality Weekly Report. 2007;56(12):276-277.

[34] Khairallah M., Kahloun R. Ocular manifestations of emerging infectious diseases. Current Opinion in Ophthalmology. 2013;24(6):574-580. DOI: 10.1097/ICU.0b013e3283654e09.

[35] Duffy M.R., Chen T., Hancock W.T., Powers A.M., Kool J.L., Lanciotti L.S., et al. Zika virus outbreak on Yap Island, Federated States of Micronesia. New England Journal of Medicine. 2009;360(24):2536-2543.

[36] Hayes, E. B. Zika virus outside Africa. Emerging Infectious Diseases. 2009;15(9): 1347-50. DOI: 10.3201/eid1509.090442.

[37] Ng A.W., Teon S.C. Dengue eye disease. Survey of Ophthalmology. 2015;60(2): 106-114. DOI: 10.1016/j.survophthal.2014.07.003.

[38] Mahendradas P., Shetty R., Narayana K.M., Shetty B.K. In vivo confocal microscopy of keratic precipitates in infectious versus noninfectious uveitis. Ophthalmology. 2010;117(2):373-380. DOI: 10.1016/j.ophtha.2009.07.016.

[39] Kanski J.J., Bowling B. Uveitis. In: Clinical Ophthalmology. A Systematic Approach. 7th ed. Elsevier España; 2011. pp. 401-471.

[40] Nalcacioglu-Yüksekkaya P., Ozdal P.C., Teke M.Y., Kara C., Ozturk F. Presumed herpetic anterior uveitis: a study with retrospective analysis of 79 cases. European Journal of Ophthalmology. 2014;24(1):14-20. DOI: 10.5301/ejo.5000331.

[41] Mittal A., Mittal S., Bharathi J.M., Ramakrishnan R., Sathe P.S. Uveitis during outbreak of chikungunya fever. Ophthalmology. 2007;114(9):1798.

[42] Jimenez-Canizales C.E., Medina-Gaitan D.A., Mondragon-Cardona A.E., Rodriguez-Morales A.J. Letter to editor: from imported to an endemic disease: impact of chikungunya virus disease in the hospital epidemiology, Tolima, Colombia, 2014-2015. Recent Patents on Anti-Infective Drug Discovery. 2015;10(1):64-66.

[43] Rodriguez-Morales A.J., Cardenas-Giraldo E.V., Montoya-Arias C.P., Guerrero-Matituy E.A., Bedoya-Arias J.E., Ramirez-Jaramillo V., et al. Mapping chikungunya fever in municipalities of one coastal department of Colombia (Sucre) using geographic in-

formation system (GIS) during 2014 outbreak: implications for travel advice. Travel Medicine and Infectious Disease. 2015;13(3):256-258. DOI: 10.1016/j.tmaid. 2015.05.007.

[44] Babu K., Murthy G.J. Chikungunya virus iridocyclitis in Fuchs' heterochromic iridocyclitis. Indian Journal of Ophthalmology. 2012;60(1):73-74. DOI: 10.4103/0301-4738.90495.

[45] Jabs D.A., Nussenblatt R.B., Rosenbaum J.T. Standardization of Uveitis Nomenclature (SUN) Working Group: standardization of uveitis nomenclature for reporting clinical data. Results of the first international workshop. American Journal of Ophthalmology. 2005;140:509-516.

[46] Sudharshan S., Ganesh S.K., Biswas J. Current approach in the diagnosis and management of posterior uveitis. Indian Journal of Ophthalmology. 2010;58(1):29-43. DOI: 10.4103/0301-4738.58470.

[47] Murthy K.R., Venkataraman N., Satish V., Babu K. Bilateral retinitis following chikungunya fever. Indian Journal of Ophthalmology. 2008;56(4):329-331.

[48] Khairallah M., Kahloun R., Yahia S.B., Jelliti B., Messaoud R. New infectious etiologies for posterior uveitis. Ophthalmic Research. 2013;49(2):66-72. DOI: 10.1159/000344009.

[49] Vishwanath S., Badami K., Sriprakash K.S., Sujatha B.L., Shashidhar S.D., Shilpa Y.D. Post-fever retinitis: a single center experience from south India. International Ophthalmology. 2014;34(4):851-857. DOI: 10.1007/s10792-013-9891-7.

[50] Shukla J., Saxena D., Rathinam S., Lalitha P., Joseph C.R., Sharma S., et al. Molecular detection and characterization of West Nile virus associated with multifocal retinitis in patients from southern India. International Journal of Infectious Diseases. 2012;16(1):53-59. DOI: 10.1016/j.ijid.2011.09.020.

[51] Sivakumar R.R., Prajna L., Arya L.K., Muraly P., Shukla J., Saxena D., et al. Molecular diagnosis and ocular imaging of West Nile virus retinitis and neuroretinitis. Ophthalmology. 2013;120(9):1820-1826. DOI: 10.1016/j.ophtha.2013.02.006.

[52] Ranjan P., Guliani B.P., Khairallah M., Mishra D. Acute necrotizing panophthalmitis in seropositive case of chikungunya: a case report and review of literature. Journal of Clinical Ophthalmology and Research. 2013;1(1):23-25..

[53] PAHO/WHO. Preparedness and Response for Chikungunya Virus: Introduction in the Americas. 2011,Washington, D.C.

[54] Khairallah M., Jelliti B., Jenzeri S. Emergent infectious uveitis. Middle East African Journal of Ophthalmology. 2009;16(4):225-238.

[55] Gupta A., Gupta V., Herbort C.P., Khairallah M. Chikungunya in uveitis. In: Uveitis: Text & Imaging. 1st ed. New Delhi: Jaypee Brothers; 2008. pp. 706-712.

Chapter 5

Dengue and Chikungunya Coinfection – The Emergence of an Underestimated Threat

Manuel Perera-Lecoin, Natthanej Luplertlop, Pornapat Surasombatpattana, Florian Liégeois, Rodolphe Hamel, Supatra Thongrungkiat, Ronald Enrique Morales Vargas, Hans Yssel and Dorothée Missé

Additional information is available at the end of the chapter

http://dx.doi.org/10.5772/64426

Abstract

Both Dengue (DENV) and Chikungunya (CHIKV) viruses can be transmitted by *Aedes* mosquito species and the diseases that they cause have several clinical symptoms in common. Co-circulation of DENV and CHIKV is increasing around the world and must therefore be considered as an emerging threat with an important public health concern. At present, very little is known about the clinical manifestations and biological consequences of coinfection by both viruses. Thus, numerous questions such as clinical severity and dynamics of viral replication of DENV and CHIKV coinfections, as well as vectorial competence, have yet to be addressed in this important and challenging research area. The ensuring knowledge will enhance the clinical surveillance and the development of diagnostic tools able to differentiate DENV and CHIKV in order to early detect virus invasion and local transmission, as well as to improve patient care and timely control measures. In this review, we highlight the current knowledge on DENV and CHIKV coinfections. We also discuss research perspectives and challenges in order to further understand the ecology and biology of this phenomenon.

Keywords: Chikungunya, Dengue, coinfection

1. Introduction

Arthropod-borne viruses represent a global threat for public health as they can be transmitted to humans by hematophagous arthropods that are rapidly spreading worldwide. These viruses belong to four major families, *Flaviviridae, Togaviridae, Rhabdoviridae, Reoviridae,* and *Bunyaviridae,* and are the etiologic agents of severe pathologies, such as yellow fever, dengue, and chikungunya diseases.

Dengue virus (DENV) is perhaps the most relevant arbovirus in terms of morbidity, mortality, and socioeconomic impact, threatening more than 2.5 billion individuals worldwide [1]. It belongs to the *Flaviviridae* family, genus *Flavivirus*, and is composed by four closely related serotypes (DENV-1, -2, -3, -4), all of which share the same icosahedral and enveloped structure with an average diameter of 50 nm. Its genome is composed of a single-stranded positive sense RNA molecule of approximately 11 kb that codifies three structural (Capsid, Membrane, and Envelope) and seven nonstructural proteins (NS1/NS2A/NS2B/NS3/NS4A/NS4B/NS5), flanked by two untranslated regions (UTRs) [2]. DENV is transmitted to humans by blood-feeding females of *Aedes* mosquitoes and, although the large majority of infections remain asymptomatic, some of them can cause a spectrum of illnesses, ranging from a flu-like disease of mild severity known as dengue fever (DF), to more severe clinical manifestations such as dengue hemorrhagic fever (DHF) that can progress to dengue shock syndrome (DSS) and death [3, 4].

Chikungunya virus (CHIKV), on the other hand, belongs to the *Togaviridae* family, genus *Alphavirus*. Like DENV, it is a small icosahedral-shaped enveloped virus approximately 70 nm in diameter. Its genome is a single-stranded positive sense RNA molecule of approximately 12 kb that contains two open reading frames (ORFs): the N-terminal ORF encodes four nonstructural proteins (nsP1 to nsP4), while its C-terminal counterpart encodes the five structural proteins C, E1, E2, E3, and 6K [5]. CHIKV is also transmitted to humans by the bite of *Aedes* mosquitoes. Clinically, infection by CHIKV is characterized by fever, headache, fatigue, rash and intense, invalidating and often persistent arthralgia that can last for years in 30–40% of infected individuals. Although rare, neurologic complications can be observed, particularly among infected neonates. The rate of mortality has been estimated to be 1 in 1000 [6, 7]. Since its first documented epidemic in 1952 in Africa, sporadic CHIKV outbreaks were reported in numerous African and Asian countries, until the virus dramatically emerged during the last decade [8]. Since then, the virus has been continuously expanding and in 2013 it reached South America and the Caribbean basin causing more than 440,000 cases of disease in more than 20 countries by mid-2014 [9, 10].

Since *Aedes* mosquitoes can be vectors of both DENV and CHIKV and as the endemic areas of these two viruses often overlap, cocirculation of DENV and CHIKV has been reported in various geographic areas, including Southeast Asia and intertropical Africa. However, despite increasing evidence showing that coinfection of humans by DENV and CHIKV is likely to be an emerging trend, very little is known about the clinical manifestations and biological consequences of this phenomenon. This represents an exciting area of research as several scientific questions remain to be answered. Are the cases of coinfection linked to the propagation of a specific species of *Aedes* mosquitoes? Can these coinfections increase the incidence of severe forms of dengue and chikungunya diseases? What are the dynamics of viral replication when both viruses infect the same cells? What are the cellular pathways that are altered upon coinfection and how do they contribute to the pathophysiology of the diseases? The current chapter will try to shed light on these interrogations by reviewing all the available data on DENV-CHIKV coinfections.

2. Epidemiology

Although similar in some aspects, the history traits and epidemiology of DENV and CHIKV have followed different patterns, both intrinsically linked to the ecology of the mosquito vectors. These topics will be reviewed individually for each virus and the cases of coinfection will be finally analyzed.

2.1. Dengue virus

2.1.1. History and epidemiology

The name dengue seems to derive from the Swahili *ki-dinga pepo*, which was employed to describe a disease characterized by cramp-like seizures. The word was introduced in the Caribbean by the slave trade from East Africa during the 1800s and progressively changed to "dengue" [11]. Dengue-associated symptoms are almost indistinguishable from those caused by other viral agents such as CHIKV, but it is generally assumed that the first reports of dengue-like illness were described in China between 269 and 992 BC. The first detailed clinical descriptions were made in the late eighteenth century by Benjamin Rush and David Bylon after epidemic episodes in Philadelphia and Indonesia, respectively [12, 13]. These cases were associated to flying insects developing in water reservoirs, but it was not until the beginning of the twentieth century that *Aedes* mosquitoes were identified as the main transmitting vectors of the virus [14, 15]. During World War II, increasing cases of dengue among the troops deployed in Africa and the Pacific led to substantial efforts to isolate the virus. Not surprisingly, the first two serotypes of DENV (DENV-1 and DENV-2) were isolated during this period in the Pacific [16]. DENV-3 and DENV-4 were discovered in the 1950s in Southeast Asia in the Philippines and Thailand [17].

Although the virus was initially thought to have originated in Africa, serological and phylogenetic studies rather point toward an Asiatic origin with a subsequent propagation to the African continent and to the Americas [18]. By analyzing the substitution rate of the Envelope (*E*) gene from DENV, it has been estimated that the origin of the virus is likely to date back to 1000 years ago and that it used primates as a reservoir [19]. The four serotypes of DENV seem to have evolved in the rainforests of Southeast Asia and cross-species transmission to humans have occurred independently in all four serotypes between 125 and 320 years ago for DENV-1 and DENV-2, respectively [3, 19, 20]. According to the results from sequence analysis of the junction of the *E* and *NS1* genes, the DENV-1 serotype has been further divided in five genotypes (I–V), while the same analysis of the *E* and *M* genes classifies DENV-3 isolates into four genotypes. DENV-2 and DENV-4 are conformed by five and three genotypes, respectively [18].

It is believed that the sylvatic forms of DENV have caused sporadic and accidental outbreaks in humans, essentially among rural communities. The burden of dengue disease seems to be linked to the widespread colonization of the tropics by *Aedes aegypti*, a species that is highly permissive to DENV and exhibits an anthropophilic behavior, thereby mediating an efficient interhuman transmission. Originally from West Africa, where it acquired its urban preference,

Ae. aegypti may have been introduced in the Americas and Asia by sailing ships, creating the ideal conditions for the spread of the disease worldwide [21]. Indeed, until the 1970s, less than 100,000 cases of dengue, diagnosed by febrile illness and hemorrhagic manifestations were registered yearly, and DHF was documented only in a dozen of countries. Furthermore, concomitant circulation of more than one serotype of DENV in a geographic region, known as hyperendemicity, was restrained to Central America, Southeast Asia, and West Africa. Thirty years later, DENV had become hyperendemic in all continents, except Antarctica, and was responsible for more than 500,000 cases of DHF and DSS reported in almost 60 countries [22]. It has been estimated that 2.5 billion individuals are at risk of infection, especially in the Americas and Asia. Recent investigations estimate to 390 million the number of DENV infections per year worldwide, leading to 96 million symptomatic dengue cases [1]. Several factors may explain the worldwide emergence of DENV. The most important one is the demographic burden observed after World War II that led to the occupation of ecological niches where the virus was circulating [18]. Unplanned urbanization with inadequate waste management and water distribution systems have facilitated the development of *Ae. aegypti* mosquitoes in densely populated areas. The increased circulation of people and merchandise has also allowed the concomitant spread of both the virus and its vectors to new geographical areas [22, 23]. Furthermore, the lack of continuity in programs aimed to eradicate the mosquitoes by massive fumigation, allowed the resurgence of *Aedes* populations in areas that were almost freed from them, particularly in South America [24].

2.1.2. Transmission and vector competence

Two main cycles of transmission have been described for DENV (Figure 1). The primitive sylvatic enzootic transmission, in Asia and Africa, involves *Aedes* spp. as vectors and lower primates as reservoirs. Occasionally, blood-feeding females of *Aedes* mosquitoes may transmit DENV to rural human communities, but these are considered as accidental contacts [3]. The urban cycle is the most relevant and challenging type of transmission, being responsible for the emergence of dengue during the twentieth century. Indeed, DENV can be maintained in a mosquito-human-mosquito cycle in urban areas, having lost the dependency on an enzootic cycle for transmission [22]. The urban cycle involves essentially *Ae. aegypti* as a vector, since this mosquito has been shown to be highly anthropophilic. This species feeds almost exclusively on human blood as a protein source for egg development [25–27]. Furthermore, *Ae. aegypti* prefers to lay its eggs in artificial water containers such as used tires, cisternae and flower pots that surround human habitats, thereby transmitting the virus transovarially to its progeny [28, 29]. It also feeds on multiple human hosts during a single gonotrophic cycle, resting indoors after the blood meal. This behavior ideally contributes to sustain the urban cyle of transmission as it increases the probability of becoming infected and transmitting the virus to multiple hosts [27].

Other species, such as *Ae. polynesiensis* and *Ae. albopictus* may also account, although as yet to a lesser extent, for the DENV urban cycle of transmission. In that sense, an increasing attention has been paid to the role of *Ae. albopictus* in the spread of DENV worldwide. This species is currently the most invasive mosquito in the world [30] and several vector competence experiments performed under laboratory conditions have shown that *Ae. albopictus* mosquitoes are more susceptible to DENV than *Ae. aegypti* [31–34], raising concerns over the possibility that the expansion of this vector will increase the risk of DENV spreading to new geographical areas. However, these experiments remain controversial, because conflicting results have been obtained showing that *Ae. aegypti* is more, or equally, susceptible to DENV infection than its counterpart *Ae. albopictus* [35–37]. In a very interesting paper, Lambrechts et al. [38] analyzed the relative public health importance of *Ae. albopictus* for DENV transmission, by performing a meta-analysis of reported studies that compared the oral susceptibility of *Ae. aegypti* and *Ae. albopictus* to DENV. The results revealed that although *Ae. albopictus* was more susceptible to infection than *Ae. aegypti*, as measured by midgut infection, the rate of virus dissemination to other tissues, as measured by the presence of the virus in the mosquito's head, was lower for *Ae. albopictus* [38]. Thus, according to these laboratory experiments, *Ae. albopictus* would not a represent a serious concern for DENV spread, as compared to *Ae. aegypti*, because of its lower capacity to become infectious and to act as an efficient vector. As pointed out by the authors, vector competence experiments are only one component of the natural and more complex vectorial capacity of a mosquito, which depends on other factors such as the ecology, the behavior, and the genetics of the vector and the virus. For example, it has been shown that vector competence can vary significantly among the vector subspecies: the *Ae. aegypti aegypti* subspecies, which is more anthropophilic than the *Ae. aegypti formosus* subspecies, is also more susceptible to DENV infection [39]. In addition, the DENV genotype is determinant, since *Ae. aegypti* is less susceptible to American DENV-2 genotypes than to Asian genotypes [40, 41]. Therefore, laboratory experiments of vector competence should be carefully interpreted and should be validated by entomological and ecological studies in the field. In that sense, several ecological observations indicate that the contribution of *Ae. albopictus* to the emergence of DENV should not be underestimated: (i) *Ae. albopcitus* was responsible of DENV outbreaks in areas where *Ae. aegypti* was absent or rare [26], such as Macao (China) [42] and Hawaii in 2001 [43], La Réunion Island in 2004 [44], Mauritius in 2009 [45], and Europe in 2010 when the first autochthonous dengue cases were reported in France [46] and Croatia [47]. (ii) The vector is massively and actively spreading worldwide and is, as mentioned above, considered to be one of the most invasive mosquito species in the world. Since 1979 it has colonized large areas of North, Central, and South America, Africa, Australia, and more than 20 countries in Europe [30, 48], where it has been mainly introduced through the trade of used tires [48, 49]. (iii) In contrast to *Ae. aegypti*, *Ae. albopictus* has the potential to adapt to low temperatures, allowing to colonize temperate climates with cold winters such as those found in Europe and North America. Indeed, it has been shown that immature forms of *Ae. albopictus* can develop in temperatures as low as 10ºC [50], and that some populations have a diapausing egg state, allowing them to resist cold winters with average temperatures below 0ºC [51, 52]. This capacity to resist low and adverse temperatures is linked to an increased efficiency to synthesize lipids in cold temperatures, as compared to *Ae. aegypti*, restricting this latter species to tropical and subtropical areas [53, 54]. (iv) Although it has generally been assumed that the feeding behavior of *Ae. albopictus* is opportunistic and zoophilic, mainly ingesting blood from nonhuman mammals, some studies have shown that *Ae. albopictus* mosquitoes caught in the wild preferentially feed on humans in Cameroon [55], Thailand [25], North Carolina [56], and the Andaman and Nicobar archipelago in India [26]. These results have been confirmed by laboratory host preference experiments with *Ae. albopictus* specimens from La Réunion Island [57]. This suggests that the feeding behavior of *Ae. albopictus* may be changing and switching to humans as a main source of blood, thus increasing the risk of human-to-human transmission mediated by this mosquito. (v) *Ae. albopictus* and *Ae. aegypti* are sympatric in numerous areas of the world, often sharing breeding sites and larval habitats [58–61]. This may lead to competitive interactions between two species eventually leading to the decline of one of the two. As suggested by field experiments performed in the United States [60, 62] and Brazil [63], when larvae from *Ae. albopictus* and *Ae. aegypti* compete for resources, it is *Ae. albopictus* that has a competitive advantage, giving a possible explanation to the local decline and extinction of indigenous *Ae. aegypti* populations following the introduction of *Ae. albopictus*. Altogether, these data emphasize the potential of *Ae. albopictus* to substitute *Ae. aegypti* and become the main vector of DENV.

2.2. Chikungunya virus

2.2.1. History and epidemiology

The name Chikungunya, meaning "the disease that bends up the joints" comes from the Makonde people in Tanzania, where the virus was first recognized in 1952 [64, 65]. Although arthralgia is one of the characteristic symptoms of chikungunya disease, most of the clinical manifestations are almost indistinguishable from those of Dengue. Thus, it is difficult to trace back the first epidemics of CHIKV in the literature and historical records. Nonetheless, it is generally assumed that the virus has been responsible for episodic outbreaks in Africa for several centuries before being imported to Asia and America by sailing ships during the eighteenth and nineteenth centuries [66–68].

On the basis of the phylogenetic analysis of the open reading frame of several CHIKV strains, the virus has been divided into three clades: West African (Waf), Asian, and East/Central/South African (ECSA), [69]. According to this study, the current CHIKV strains derived from a common ancestor that existed around 500 years ago. The divergence between the ECSA and the Asian clades occurred during the end of the nineteenth and the beginning of the twentieth centuries. Interestingly, despite their close geographic proximity, the ECSA and West African strains are highly divergent for reasons that are not yet completely understood. The recent Indian Ocean monophyletic lineage (IOL) originated from the ECSA group at the beginning of the twentieth century [69].

It is assumed that CHIKV originated in Africa, where it circulated in an enzootic cycle responsible for sporadic human epidemic outbreaks during the twentieth century in Tanzania in 1952 [64], Uganda in 1958 [70], South Africa in 1976 [71], Sudan in 1988 [72], and Senegal in 1996 [73], all arising from rural communities in close proximity to forested areas. However, more recent CHIKV outbreaks linked to indigenous ECSA strains have arisen in urban centers, as observed in Congo, Cameroon, and Gabon during 2000–2010 [74–76].

In Asia, the virus was first isolated in Thailand in 1958 [77] and was responsible for large epidemics affecting millions of people in Sri Lanka and India between 1963 and 1973, when the last CHIKV epidemic was recorded in 2005 [78–80]. This year marks the reemergence of CHIKV on the Indian subcontinent with the introduction of the IOL coming from islands in the Indian Ocean [80–82]. Indeed, after its initial detection in Kenya in 2004 [83], IOL subsequently spread to these islands, among which Mauritius, Comoros, Mayotte, Seychelles, La Réunion, and Madagascar, during 2005–2006 [84, 85]. The extent of the epidemics by this new strain is reflected by the example of La Réunion, where 266,000 individuals, a third of the island population, became infected, which resulted in around 260 deaths, most of them elderly people [86, 87]. After its introduction in India and Sri Lanka, the IOL CHIKV strains spread quickly throughout Southeast Asia, being responsible of outbreaks in Malaysia [88], Singapore [89], and Thailand [90] in 2008, China in 2010 [91], Cambodia in 2011 [92], and Bhutan in 2012 [93]. Overall, it is estimated that CHIKV has caused more than two million cases since 2004 in Africa and Asia [94]. IOL strains also have become a concern in Europe, where they were imported by infected travelers returning from India and were responsible for outbreaks in Italy in 2007 [95] and France in 2010 [96] and 2014 [97], both likely transmitted by resident populations of *Ae. albopictus*.

In America, the presence of CHIKV has formally been identified in 2013 in Saint Martin Island during a large and ongoing epidemic in the Caribbean basin [98], although it is suspected to be responsible for several epidemics since the nineteenth century. Since then, CHIKV has spread to the other Antilles islands where *Ae. aegypti* was the only known vector present [98]. The virus then reached Central, South, and North America, where 11 cases of local CHIKV transmission were recorded in 2014 [9]. Overall, the CHIKV burden in the Americas caused more than a 1.7 million suspected cases, with almost 60.000 confirmed cases and more than 200 deaths in the 2013–2015 period [99]. Interestingly, this epidemic burden was not initiated by the highly invasive IOL, but rather by Asian CHIKV strains [98]. These strains have maintained their endemic circulation in Asia alongside the IOL burden, provoking recent outbreaks in Indonesia and the Philippines [100, 101] as well as in the Pacific [102].

2.2.2. Transmission and vector competence

Similar to DENV, two modes of transmission have been described for CHIKV that rely on the same *Aedes* vectors (Figure 1). In Africa, CHIKV has been circulating in an enzootic cycle between forest-dwelling *Aedes* spp. mosquitoes and nonhuman primates as a reservoir [103]. This mode of transmission is believed to be the source of the sporadic and remote African Chikungunya outbreaks recorded during the twentieth century. However, increasing urbanization and the establishment of anthropophilic and peridomestic *Ae. aegypti* and *Ae. albopictus* populations, seem to be changing the dynamics of CHIKV spread in Africa, provoking larger epidemics associated with an urban cycle of transmission that relies on humans as a reservoir. This urban transmission is most likely responsible for the recent Chikungunya outbreaks in Western Africa [75, 76].

In Asia, CHIKV has traditionally circulated in an urban cycle associated with the presence of *Ae. aegypti* and *albopictus* mosquitoes. As a consequence, Asian CHIKV epidemics have been larger and have spread more rapidly than those in Africa.

Vector competence studies, (reviewed in [103]), have shown that both *Ae. aegypti* and *Ae. albopictus* are highly susceptible to CHIKV infection and are both able to transmit the virus to humans. However, the Indian Ocean epidemics have provided a very interesting case of viral adaptation to a specific vector. Indeed, during the second half of 2005, a genetic change (alanine to valine substitution) occurred at position 226 of the E1 membrane fusion glycoprotein in the viral IOL strains that were circulating in the area. This mutation was absent in the initial strains and became prevalent after its introduction, being present in more than 90% of the isolates obtained in La Réunion during 2005–2006 [104]. Further laboratory experiments showed that this mutation was directly responsible for an increase in CHIKV infectivity for *Aedes albopictus,* improving viral dissemination and the transmission to suckling mice without affecting viral fitness in *Ae. aegypti* [105, 106]. Interestingly, this mutation was acquired independently in several distinct geographical locations (India and West Africa) where, similarly to La Réunion, *Aedes albopictus* is widely present and is actively displacing indigenous *Ae. aegypti* populations. Therefore, it has been suggested that the A226V mutation is a clear example of convergent evolution, allowing CHIKV viral strains to adapt to the prevalent mosquito vector [107]. The molecular explanation for the increased fitness in *Aedes albopictus* conferred by A226V mutations has not been completely unraveled. It was initially suggested that this mutation increased the dependency on cholesterol during the virus-host cell fusion step, based on the observation that mutated CHIKV isolates showed an attenuated viral growth in C6/36 mosquito cells devoid of cholesterol, as compared to original, nonmutated, strains [6, 105]. Therefore, it was suspected that this differential phenotype was responsible for the preferential replication in *Aedes albopictus* mosquitoes. However, further studies revealed that there is no a clear correlation between the dependence on cholesterol and capacity of the virus to infect *Ae. albopictus,* suggesting that these are two independent phenotypic effects of the E1 226 mutation [108]. Interestingly, second-step adaptative mutations have been described in A226V CHIKV strains that further potentiate viral replication in *Ae. albopictus*. One of these consists in a leucine for glutamine substitution in position 210 (L210Q) of the E2 protein that mediates viral binding. This mutation, characterized in viral isolates from Kerala in Southwest India [109], facilitates infection of midgut epithelial mosquito cells, thereby increasing viral dissemination and transmission by *Aedes albopictus* without a significant effect on *Ae. aegypti* [110]. Altogether, these data demonstrate that some CHIKV strains are rapidly evolving to exploit *Aedes albopictus* as a major vector in areas where it is abundant, raising concern about the epidemic potential of these strains in the Europe and North America where the mosquito is rapidly spreading.

Another interesting observation is that A226V mutation appeared in ECSA CHIKV strains and not in the Asian strains circulating in areas where *Aedes albopictus* is common [111]. This phenomenon has been attributed to evolutionary constraints imposed by epistatic interactions between residues 226 and 98 of the E1 glycoprotein. Indeed, all endemic Asian strains have a threonine in position 98 that is absent in both IOL and ECSA strains and that limits the adaptative effect of the A226V mutation in *Aedes albopictus* [111]. This constraint is likely to guarantee that the ongoing American CHIKV epidemics, caused by Asian strains, will be sustained by *Ae. aegypti* instead of *Ae. albopictus* in areas where they are sympatric [103]. However, this dynamic may change if introduced *Ae. albopictus*-fitted ECSA and IOL strains settle in the area.

In addition, a recent experimental study conducted by Stapleford et al. [112] showed the emergence of two new mutations V80I and 129V on E1 glycoprotein of the CHIKV A226V strain. Positive selection of these mutations appears to improve the stability and fusogenic activity of these variants. This study offers an interesting predictive approach to guide the monitoring of CHIKV strains involved in future outbreaks [112].

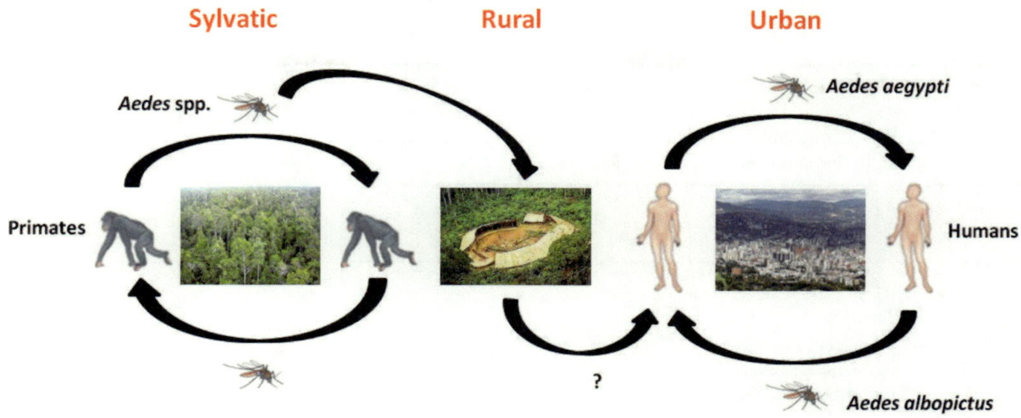

Figure 1. Transmission cycles of DENV and CHIKV. In the sylvatic cycle, primate hosts and several species of *Aedes* mosquitoes sustain DENV and CHIKV transmission. Occasionally, rural communities surrounding forests can become infected. The urban cycle of transmission may have been initiated by the migration of infected individuals from those rural communities to the cities. The urban cycle involves essentially *Ae. aegypti and Aedes albopictus* as vectors and humans as reservoirs. Adapted from [113–115].

2.3. DENV-CHIKV coinfections

2.3.1. History of reported cases

To date, the number of diagnosed cases of DENV-CHIKV coinfections is surprisingly small and available information is often incomplete, making it difficult to establish epidemiological trends. However, it is noteworthy that the number of reported cases has increased considerably during the past 10 years (Table 1, Figure 2), indicating that the phenomenon is becoming a concern among the scientific community because of its potential impact on human health and economy. Indeed, although the first documented cases of DENV-CHIKV coinfections date back to the 1960s in Vellore, South India, when 14 cases were reported during a CHIKV epidemic outbreak [116, 117], and in Thailand [118], where nine cases were documented, it was not until 2006 that the diagnosis of concomitant infections experienced a real interest, possibly due to the burden of cases of chikungunya infection in the Indian Ocean's island and Southeast Asia where DENV is endemic.

In 2006, two cases of coinfection corresponding to two female patients were described in Malaysia, and 20 more were recorded during the CHIKV outbreak in La Réunion the same year. More cases of coinfection were reported in Madagascar and Sri Lanka in 2006–2007 and in Gabon, India, Nigeria and Singapore during 2007–2010, coinciding with the epidemics of CHIKV caused by IOL strains during this period in the area. The most recent cases were diagnosed in South America, India and Nigeria in 2013–2014. Of note, two of these cases corresponded to infected travelers returning to Portugal and Germany after being infected in Angola and India, respectively [119,120], raising concern about the possible spread of coinfection cases in Europe where *Aedes albopictus* is present.

Number of cases	Location	Year	DENV serotype	CHIKV clade			Severe symptoms	Vector	Reference
				Asian	ECSA	Waf			
9	Thailand	1962-1964	NS[a]		NS		NS	NS	[118]
14	Vellore, India	1964	DENV-2		NS		Absence	NS	[116, 117]
20	La Réunion	2005-2006	NS		X		NS	NS	[121]
2	Kinta District, Malaysia	2006	DENV-1		X		1 case of DHF	NS	[122]
10	Toamasina, Madagascar	2006	DENV-1		NS		Absence	*Ae. albopictus*	[123]
3	Kandy, Sri Lanka	2006-2007	NS		NS		1 case with Guillain barré syndrome	NS	[82]
37	Gabon	2007-2010	DENV-2		X		Absence	*Ae. albopictus*	[124, 125]
1	Chennai, India	2008	NS	NS			Absence	NS	[119]
63	Nigeria	2008	NS				Absence	NS	[126]
6	Delhi, India	2009	DENV-3 DENV-4 DENV-3/4 DENV-1/4		X		2 DHF, 1 dead	NS	[127]
1	Singapore	2009	DENV-2		X		Absence	NS	[128]
43	Maharashtra and Odisha, India	2013	DENV-2 DENV-1 DENV-3		X		3 cases of DHF	NS	[129]
16	Saint Martin	2013-2014	DENV-1 DENV-2 DENV-4	X			Absence	*Ae. aegypti*	[130]
1	Nigeria	2014	NS	NS			Absence	NS	[131]
1	Luanda, Angola	2014	DENV-4		X		Absence	NS	[120]
2	India	NS	NS	NS			Absence	NS	[132]

Table 1. Reported cases of DENV/CHIKV coinfections. [a] NS: Not specified.

As shown in Table 1, the four serotypes of DENV can be found in association with both the Asian and ECSA CHIKV clades, depending of the strain of CHIKV that cocirculates with

DENV in a particular area, pertaining to Asian CHIKV strains in America and ECSA strains in Asia and Africa. However, it would be interesting to study if some particular associations of DENV and CHIKV genotypes are favored in nature. For example, is the circulation of some virulent DENV strains associated with the simultaneous presence of specific CHIKV genotypes? Such preferential associations could provide insight into viral coevolution and allow to define strategies to limit the morbidity associated with certain highly pathogenic viral strains.

2.3.2. Transmission and vector competence

Some of the studies reported in Table 1 provide interesting information about the relative importance of *Aedes albopictus* and *Ae. aegypti* in the spread of coinfection cases in natural conditions. Perhaps the most complete and documented cases of coinfection from an epidemiological perspective have been provided by a large clinical, virological, and entomological study performed in Gabon between 2007 and 2010 [124, 125]. During this period, an active surveillance of acute febrile symptoms was implemented in the healthcare centers of Libreville and all the major towns of the country. Blood was sampled from patients who met the case definition for diagnosis of CHIKV and DENV infection, as determined by quantitative PCR [124, 125]. A total of 4287 patients were tested among which 1567 (36.6% of the individuals) were CHIKV-positive, 376 (8.3%) were DENV-2 positive (no other serotype was reported) and 37 (0.9%) were coinfected with both viruses. All cases occurred in densely populated areas during the rainy season, when conditions are ideal for mosquito breeding. Two large epidemic outbreaks were observed, during 2007 and 2010, with sporadic cases in between. In 2007, the vast majority of CHIKV and DENV-2 infections were reported around the capital Libreville, in the Northwest, with nine cases of coinfection. During 2008 and 2009, the viruses moved to Lambaréné, Ndjolé, and Lastourville in the center and the south of the country, respectively, however no cases of coinfection were reported. Finally, the 2010 outbreak occurred in the southeast of the country and was centered around Franceville, close to the Congo border where 28 cases of coinfected patients were recorded. The phylogenetic study, based on the isolates recovered from monoinfected and coinfected patients not only showed that CHIKV belonged to the ECSA lineage, but also that the Gabonese strains from 2010 derived from those reported in 2007, which were in turn closely related to the CHIKV strains isolated in 2006 from an outbreak in Cameroon [74]. These findings suggest that CHIKV is spreading rapidly in Western Central Africa with a north to south dynamic, a trend that seems to be confirmed by the identification of the virus in Southern Congo in 2011 [133] and Angola in 2014 [120]. On the other hand, DENV-2 isolates from 2010 also derived from those of 2007 and were found to cluster in the cosmopolitan genotype, which gathers strains isolated in diverse areas of the world such as India, China, Australia, and Saudi Arabia. The most likely explanation for these observations is that the DENV-2 Gabonese strains were imported by infected travelers coming from the latter areas or by infected mosquitoes introduced in Gabon along with imported products [124, 125].

During this study, mosquitoes were captured around the coinfected patient's homes. After identification of the species, viral presence was determined by quantitative PCR from pooled mosquitoes abdomen. In total, 661 *Aedes* mosquitoes were analyzed. A large majority of the

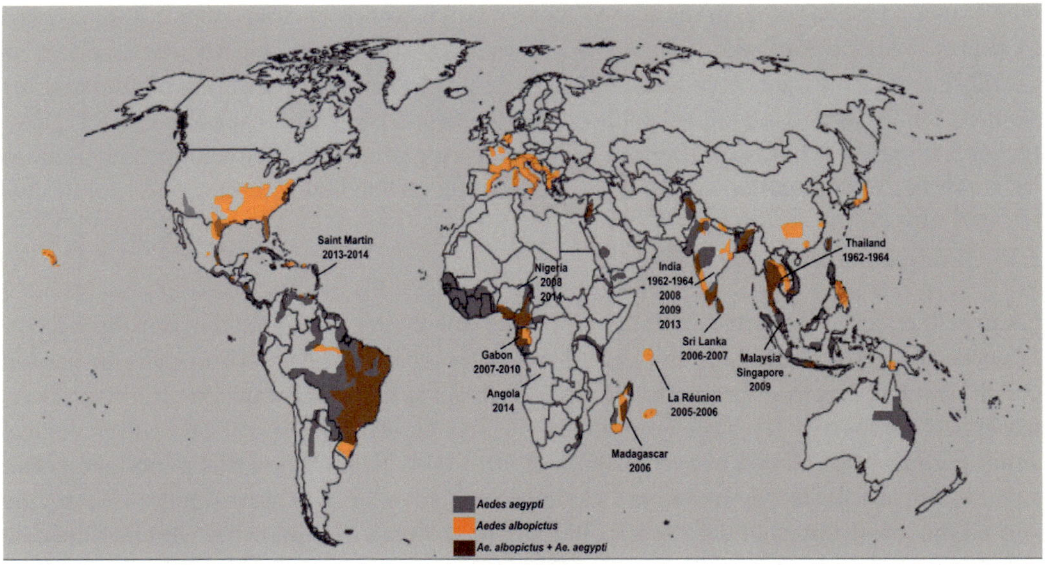

Figure 2. Geographical distribution of *Aedes albopictus* and *Aedes aegypti* populations and locations where DENV/CHIKV coinfections have been described. Adapted from [134].

mosquitoes was constituted by *Ae. albopictus* (571 specimens, 86% of the caught specimens), followed by *Ae. simpsoni* and *Ae. aegypti* (52 and 38 specimens, respectively). From the 46 pooled abdomens of *Ae. albopictus* 11 (23.9% of total) tested positive for CHIKV, 18 (39.1%) for DENV-2 and three (6.5%) for both viruses. This was the first report of a concomitant infection of mosquitoes by CHIKV and DENV in nature. In the case of *Ae. aegypti*, one out of the three pools (33.3%) tested positive for CHIKV, whereas DENV-2 was not detected. All three *Ae. simpsoni* pools tested negative for both viruses. Although the lack of detection of both viruses in *Ae. aegypti* specimens could be attributed to the large predominance of *Ae. albopictus*, which increases the probability of the latter vector to be coinfected, another study comparing the roles of the two species in the emergence of DENV and CHIKV in central Africa confirmed that the only species naturally infected by DENV and CHIKV was *Ae. albopictus* [135]. This is not surprising with respect to CHIKV, because the viral isolates circulating in the area have acquired the A226V substitution and are therefore particularly adapted to grow in *Ae. albopictus* [107, 125]. The absence of *Ae. aegypti*, naturally infected with DENV, has been attributed to the poor susceptibility of this mosquito to DENV in this region, explaining the lack of DENV outbreaks in West and Central Africa until the turn of the century with the introduction of *Ae. albopictus* [39]. This notion has been confirmed by laboratory experiments showing that *Ae. aegypti* specimens collected from Cameroon are less susceptible to DENV infection than mosquitoes of Asia and South America [135].

Besides its greater susceptibility to CHIKV and DENV, *Ae. albopictus* may be more efficient in the maintenance of DENV and CHIKV transmission cycles because of its aggressive feeding behavior, with a human biting rate that is significantly higher than the one observed in *Ae. aegypti* populations in suburban areas of Central Africa, according to a study led by Paupy et al. [135]. This may increase the probability of *Ae. albopictus* mosquitoes of becoming infected by DENV and CHIKV and transmitting the viruses to human hosts.

These data indicate that *Ae. albopictus* is more fitted to transmit both viruses and to act as the primary vector of DENV and CHIKV in Gabon which should raise concerns about the spread of CHIKV/DENV coinfections to the rest of Africa in view of the continuing progression of *Ae. albopictus* on this continent.

The disproportion in the abundance of *Aedes* species in Gabon is striking as *Ae. albopictus* was first reported in the country in 2006 [136, 137], suggesting that the species is rapidly proliferating and actively displacing endemic populations of *Ae. aegypti*. This trend has been confirmed by a subsequent entomological study carried in different locations of Gabon, demonstrating that *Ae. albopictus* largely outnumbered the endemic *Ae. aegypti* populations in suburban areas where patches of vegetation are likely to be present, as well as in small towns particularly affected by the 2007–2010 DENV/CHIKV epidemics such as Cocobeach, Oyem, and Lastourville [135].

This trend and the role of *Ae. albopictus* as the main vector of CHIKV/DENV coinfections were confirmed by Ratsitorahina et al. who conducted a virologic and entomologic study in the city of Toamasina, located in the eastern coast of Madagascar, following an outbreak of dengue-like symptoms (DLS) [123]. CHIKV was suspected as the etiologic agent, because the virus was previously detected in La Réunion, the Seychelles, and Comoros archipelagos during the IOL CHIKV epidemic. Blood samples were taken from 55 febrile patients manifesting headache, myalgia, arthralgia, retroorbital pain, or rash. Molecular and serological diagnostics identified CHIKV (IO lineage, highly adapted to *Ae. albopictus*) and DENV-1 (closely related to strains isolated in La Réunion in 2004) in 38 of the 55 patients, among which 10 cases corresponded to coinfections. An entomologic study was performed in five neighborhoods in which DLS were reported, by catching mosquitoes larvae and adults in potential breeding sites. *Ae. albopictus*, a species that has been circulating in Madagascar since the 1970s [58], was the only urban vector of DENV and CHIKV and no other species were identified. Among all the mosquito pools tested for the presence of CHIKV and DENV, 21.7% tested positive for CHIKV. Data for DENV was not given. The identification of the breeding sites revealed that populations of *Ae. albopictus* from Toamasina exploit diverse artificial peridomestic containers such as tires, coconut shells, discarded cans, pots, etc., which are traditionally associated with *Ae. aegypti* populations. This highlights the notion that *Ae. albopictus* is able to adapt to the ecological niches found in urban areas and therefore could replace *Ae. aegypti* as the main vector of the urban transmission cycle of DENV and CHIKV. Accordingly, a large entomologic survey carried in 15 sites across Madagascar during the 2007–2009 period, revealed that *Ae. albopictus* has extended its geographical distribution on the island and that its population density has become consequently higher than that of *Ae. aegypti*, a species that is becoming rare. This contrasting result to what was previously reported in the 1970s–1980s, can be explained by the environmental plasticity of this species that exhibits a greater capacity to adapt to different climatic conditions and to anthropogenic changes in the natural habitats, as compared to *Ae. aegypti* [58].

Vector competence studies performed in laboratory conditions have shown that *Ae. albopictus* specimens from La Réunion are able to disseminate DENV and CHIKV and to deliver both infectious particles concomitantly in its saliva after being orally exposed to DENV and CHIKV strains, circulating in the island during 2004–2006 [138]. Another study revealed that *Ae. aegypti,* orally fed with CHIKV and DENV, is unable to sustain dual infection [139]. Although these results should be interpreted with caution since vector susceptibility is highly dependent on the origin of *Aedes* specimens, as well as the type of CHIKV and DENV strains involved in the infection, they corroborate what has already been shown in natural conditions and furthermore confirm the potential of *Ae. albopictus* to transmit both viruses more efficiently than *Ae. aegypti.*

Taken together, these results reveal an important and threatening role of *Ae. albopictus* through its ability to concomitantly transmit DENV and CHIKV in areas where it circulates sympatrically with *Ae. aegypti.* It is to be noted however, that in locations where *Ae. albopictus* is still absent, *Ae. aegypti* can sustain the concomitant transmission of both viruses, as recently reported during the Caribbean CHIKV outbreak. This epidemic that initiated in Saint Martin then spread to the French Antilles, causing a total 570 confirmed cases of infection with the Asian strain of CHIKV, 65 with DENV and 16 cases of coinfection (Table 1) [130]. *Ae. aegypti* was identified as the unique potential vector of this outbreak [98]. Nonetheless, because of the rapid propagation of *Ae. albopictus* in South America, this dynamic may change in a close future.

Another important topic related to CHIKV/DENV coinfections, is the mode by which these viruses can be transmitted to humans. Two main possibilities could be envisaged: an individual transmission of each virus by different monoinfected mosquitoes or concomitant transmission by a coinfected vector. In that sense, the study performed by Caron et al. [124] gives several interesting clues based on the analysis of viral loads detected in coinfected Gabonese patients. The results revealed the presence of two distinctive groups of patients, based on the presence of viral RNA-derived complementary DNA (cDNA): one group with a high DENV-2 cDNA load and low CHIKV cDNA load and the other with high cDNA levels of both viruses. According to this pattern of infection, the authors suggested two different modes of transmission. In patients with the highest DENV-2 cDNA, the blood samples were most likely taken during the acute phase of DENV infection and the early or late stage of CHIKV infection, suggesting that the viruses were more likely to have been transmitted by the bite of two different mosquitoes each infected with one virus, although with several days of interval, which might explain the gap between the replication kinetics of either virus. However this interpretation should be taken with caution, as several other possibilities may exist. For example, both viruses could have been transmitted by the same mosquito and DENV-2 might have replicated more efficiently than CHIKV due to genetic factors intrinsic to the human host, thus establishing a competitive state in which CHIKV could have been disadvantaged. Alternatively, DENV-2 viral load in the coinfected mosquito salivary glands may have largely exceeded that of CHIKV. As a result, the number of DENV viral particles transmitted to the human host during the mosquito bite may have been higher than for CHIKV, consequently explaining the difference in the observed cDNA loads. Another possibility, noted by Caron et al. [124], is that the immune response against DENV may have limited the replication of CHIKV. In the second group of patients with high cDNA loads for both viruses, indicative of a blood sample taken during the acute phase of both CHIKV and DENV-2 infections, the dual infection may have resulted from two rapidly succeeding bites of different mosquitoes, each infected by one virus or from the bite of a single coinfected mosquito [124].

3. Pathogenesis

From a public health perspective, the concern about coinfections is their possible impact on the pathogenesis and the outcome of dengue and chikungunya diseases. Is there a correlation between the cases of coinfection and the severity of symptoms? Because, in terms of morbidity, severity and mortality DENV has a higher impact on human health than CHIKV, the major preoccupation is that CHIKV/DENV coinfection could increase the incidence of DHF and DSS.

DHF symptoms appear around the time of defervescence, 3–7 days after the first symptoms of DF. It is characterized by an increase in capillary permeability with a loss of plasma volume that is preceded by thrombocytopenia and leukopenia. Hamorrhagic symptoms include petechiae, ecchymoses, and purpuric lesions. If a critical volume of plasma is lost through leakage, DSS may follow. This phase is characterized by a narrow pulse pressure that can be underestimated as most of the patients remain conscious and lucid. Prolonged hypotensive shock and hypoxia may result in organ failure, acidosis, intravascular coagulation, and death if not corrected in time [3, 4].

Although the pathogenesis of DENV infection is not well understood, several risk factors may increase the severity of the disease: the viral genotype (the Asian genotype of DENV-2 is considered to be a virulent strain), the age (children are less able to compensate plasma leakage than adults), the ethnicity (Caucasian are more susceptible to develop severe forms of the disease), chronic diseases (individuals with allergies, asthma, and diabetes are at higher risk than healthy people) and secondary infection with a new DENV serotype [140–143]. The latter issue has received particular attention, because it may be a major determinant for the development of severe cases of dengue. Indeed, when preexisting antibodies from a primary DENV infection bind to an infecting DENV particle during a subsequent infection with a different dengue serotype, the antibodies from the primary infection cannot neutralize the virus. Instead, the resulting antibody-virus complexes attach to Fc receptors at the surface of monocytes, macrophages, and dendritic cells (DCs), resulting in increased infection [113, 144, 145]. This phenomenon, known as antibody-dependent enhancement of infection (ADE), may explain the higher viremia and levels of circulating antigens detected in patients with DHF as compared to patients with DF [146, 147]. ADE accounts for the particular propensity of populations living in DENV hyperendemic regions to develop severe forms of dengue. ADE may also contribute to increased capillary permeability and to a "cytokine storm" that could aggravate the disease [148–150]. Another phenomenon increasing the risk of severe disease during secondary infections with DENV is the original antigenic sin or Hoskins effect. This effect refers to the tendency of the immune system to respond to a secondary infection through the activation of memory B and T cells induced by the primary infection. These cells show a decreased affinity for secondary antigens and are less effective in the control of the infection [151]. In particular, it has been shown that during the secondary infection by a different strain of dengue virus, the cytotoxic T lymphocytes release cytokines, rather than causing the lysis of infected cells, thereby increasing vascular permeability and exacerbating the damage of endothelial cells [152]. Taken together these data indicate that secondary heterotypic infections with DENV are an important factor in the aggravation of dengue disease.

However, despite the identification of risk factors, little attention has been paid to the potential effect of the simultaneous presence of CHIKV on the propensity to develop DHF. To date, the scarcely available clinical data about coinfections impedes to establish clear conclusions. The large majority of the studies analyzing the clinical symptoms of CHIKV/DENV coinfected patients failed to identify a particular predisposition to develop DHF, as no severe symptoms were observed (Table 1). Furthermore, two studies that compared the biological and clinical symptoms between monoinfected and coinfected patients did not observe more severe manifestations or biological disorders in patients with a mixed infection, suggesting that the two viruses do not exert additive effects [124, 153].

The rare cases of DHF in coinfected patients were observed in one of the two patients coinfected in Malaysia [122] and in India in 2009 [127]. The latter case deserves further attention: during this episode of DENV/CHIKV coinfections in Delhi, 69 blood samples were taken from patients with acute fever. Forty-eight were DENV-positive, eleven tested positive for ECSA lineage and six were positive for both viruses. From these six samples, three were positive for DENV-3, one for DENV-4, one for DENV-3/DENV-4 and one for DENV-1/DENV-4, constituting the first cases of concomitant infections with multiple DENV serotypes in CHIKV/DENV infected patients. Two of the six patients manifested severe hamorrhagic symptoms with central nervous system involvement and one died. It was not specified whether the severe cases corresponded to patients infected with a single DENV serotype or with two different serotypes, making it difficult to link the severity of the disease to the concomitant presence of CHIKV or to the presence of two different DENV serotypes. However, the particular high incidence of severe symptoms following superinfection by CHIKV and several DENV serotypes highlights the potential threat of CHIKV infection to human health in areas where DENV is hyperendemic [127].

Overall, these results do not establish a clear association between the severity of dengue and chikungunya diseases and the concomitant presence of both viruses. However, the number of CHIKV/DENV coinfections reported to the date is too small to draw firm conclusions. Further studies need to be undertaken with large cohorts of infected patients to gain better insight in this process, particularly taking into account that many severe cases associated with coinfections may have passed unnoticed, as the diagnosis of both viruses has not systematically been undertaken in the past. Moreover, the increase in coinfections with both viruses could lead to a rapid viral evolution, potentially resulting in the appearance of highly infective and pathogenic CHIKV and DENV strains.

4. Cell biology of CHIKV/DENV coinfections

Very little is known about the interactions that are established by the viruses and their host cells during coinfections. The fact that viral RNA of both viruses has been detected in *Aedes* abdomens strongly suggests that they can disseminate and coexist simultaneously in these mosquitoes. Accordingly, both viruses are able to concomitantly infect *Ae. aegypti* midgut and upregulate the expression of proteins involved in the oxidative stress, energy production, and carbohydrate/lipid metabolism. This shows that CHIKV and DENV are able to simultaneously circumvent the physical barrier established by the midgut to propagate to other *Aedes* organs and tissues [154]. However, almost nothing has been described at the cellular level: to date, only one work addressed the concomitant effect of CHIKV/DENV infection in mosquito cells but no information is able regarding vertebrate cells.

In this study, Potiwat et al. [155] infected *Ae. albopictus* C6/36 cells with different multiplicities of infection (MOIs) of CHIKV (ECSA strain) and DENV-3 isolates from Southern Thailand, detecting the presence of viral RNA in cell culture medium by RT-PCR. They observed that both viruses were able to replicate and generate viral progeny when cells were challenged simultaneously with a mixed viral preparation in which the viruses were added at the same MOI. However, when the proportion of viral input was changed and the titer of DENV largely exceeded the one of CHIKV, DENV was able to suppress CHIKV replication. The reciprocal (larger titer of CHIKV than DENV) did not exert any effect on DENV replication. When infection by each virus was performed sequentially at the same titer (superinfection conditions in which one virus was added 1 hour before the other), viral progeny was detected for the two viruses independently of the order of infection. Although these experiments were not validated with other viral strains and mosquito cells, they provide the first cell biology evidence that both viruses can replicate actively in the same cells when these are challenged simultaneously or sequentially. This supports the two modes of mosquito coinfection that have been suggested to occur in natural conditions: a mosquito could get coinfected by ingesting its blood meal from a viremic individual carrying both viruses, or sequentially by ingesting the blood from two different individuals each infected by a single virus. When the blood meal is taken from a single individual, the successful replication of both viruses in mosquitoes may require some conditions to be fulfilled, such as the presence of enough infectious CHIKV/DENV particles in a proportion that falls within a certain range. In other words, the quantity of one of the viral species should not overwhelmingly exceed the other one to avoid any competitive suppression. In that sense, a very recent study performed by Nuckols et al. [156] seems to confirm *in vivo* what is observed at the cellular level. In this work, *Ae. aegypti* and *Ae. albopictus* mosquitoes were challenged either simultaneously or sequentially with CHIKV and DENV-2 mixed in blood meals. After mosquito sacrifice, viral dissemination and transmission potential were assessed by detecting CHIKV and DENV RNA in the mosquito's head and saliva, respectively. The results show that both *Aedes* species exhibited a dual disseminated infection when viruses were administered at the same time or sequentially. However, CHIKV and DENV were only detected concomitantly in mosquito's saliva from specimens exposed to each virus sequentially and not simultaneously. Thus, this laboratory experiments suggest that *Aedes* mosquitoes are able to transmit both viruses to vertebrate hosts when they acquire

CHIKV and DENV with a time interval and that simultaneous acquisition of both viruses may generate competitive interactions that decrease their potential transmission. Although in this study the viral titers of DENV (3.2×10^6 focus forming units/mL) and CHIKV (1.5×10^5 plaque forming units) used to infect the mosquitoes were not comparable, it would have been interesting to assess if the competitive exclusion was due to the excess of one viral species over the other one or if it could be seen independently of the viral input.

In the work of Potiwat et al. [155], competitive suppression was only observed when the amount of viral particles from DENV largely exceeded the one from CHIKV and not the reciprocal. Both viruses are able to exploit similar cell surface receptors for attachment, such as prohibitin and heat shock proteins that can be found in mosquito cells [157–160], leading to possible competitive interactions between both viruses for attachment and viral entry. However, it is highly unlikely that this is the reason for the suppression of CHIKV replication by DENV, as no inhibition of DENV replication was observed when CHIKV particles outnumbered DENV particles, as it would be expected if the viruses rely on the same receptors for infectious entry. An alternative, is that the viruses are able to exploit different receptors on the same cell, and that an excess in DENV particles attached to the cell surface sterically interfere with CHIKV-receptors interactions. Another possibility is that the excessive entry of infectious DENV particles leads to the hijacking of cellular components necessary for CHIKV replication, or to the production of viral components that inhibit CHIKV infection.

There is no information about the cellular biology of CHIKV/DENV coinfection in mammalian cells and we can only speculate about the possible mechanisms involved in viral replication. As summarized in Table 2, CHIKV and DENV share similar mechanisms of entry, which could lead to suppressive competition between the viruses in the early steps of infection. For example, they are able to exploit similar cellular receptors for attachment, they are internalized mainly by clathrin-mediated endocytosis and their fusion occurs in the endosomal system. The cellular tropism is also similar, although it seems to be larger in the case of DENV, a phenomenon that could be explained by the longer and more frequent circulation of the virus among human beings, allowing it to adapt and exploit a more diverse range of cellular targets. However, the viral RNA of both viruses can be detected in the blood of coinfected humans, suggesting that they are both able to concomitantly invade, replicate and spread in different organs to establish a systemic infection resulting in viremia. Thus, these viruses seem to have adopted different replicative strategies to overcome the potential competition for cellular resources when they infect the same mammalian cells, and/or have established cooperative interactions to guarantee their survival and propagation in human hosts. For example, during the cellular attachment step, the viruses may use different not yet characterized receptors or use an abundant cell surface molecule to limit competition. Also, although both viruses enter cells by clathrin-mediated endocytosis, some differences exist in the pathways and molecular partners involved in the process between CHIKV and DENV. Indeed, the depletion of the fuzzy homologue (FUZ), a cytoplasmic effector protein involved in planar cell polarity, ciliogenesis, and mammalian embryonic development, strongly inhibits clathrin-mediated endocytosis of CHIKV and other alphaviruses without affecting DENV entry [161]. This suggests that both viruses exploit parallel clathrin pathways involving different effector proteins. Furthermore, DENV and CHIKV membrane fusion, a step necessary for the release of the viral genome in the cell, takes place in distinct cellular compartments: the first one occurs in $Rab7^+$ late endosomes, while the second one takes place preferentially in $Rab5^+$ early endosomes [162–164].The explanation for the selective use of these compartments could be linked to the lipidic composition of the endosomes: fusion of flaviviruses seems to require the presence of anionic lipids such as phosphatidylserine and bis(monoacylglycero)phosphate that are present in the late endosomes [165], while alphaviruses may have distinct requirements.

		DENV	CHIKV	Reference
Tropism in humans (main cell targets)	Keratinocytes	+	-	[166–172]
	Fibroblasts	+	+	
	Dendritic cells	+	-	
	Monocytes	+	-	
	Macrophages	+	+	
	Epithelial cells	+	+	
	Endothelial cells	+	+	
Attachment receptors in mammalian cells (name of the specific receptors)	Glycosaminoglycans	+	+	Reviewed in [173, 174]
	Heat Shock Proteins	+ GRP78 HSP70 HSP90	+ HSP60	
	Laminin Receptor	+	NI	
	Prohibitin	Used in mosquitoes	+	
	C-type lectins	+ DC-SIGN L-SIGN CLEC5A Mannose receptor	NI	
	Phosphatidylserine receptors	+ TIM TAM	+ TIM TAM	
	Integrins	+ Integrin $\alpha v\beta 3$	+ ITGAV ITGB1	
	Scavenger receptors	+	NI	

		DENV	CHIKV	Reference
	Claudin-1	+	NI	
	Nkp44	+	NI	
Main internalization pathway		Clathrin-dependent endocytosis	Clathrin-dependent endocytosis	[161, 164, 170, 174–179]
Compartment of viral fusion		Late endosomes	Early endosomes	[162–164]
Strategy for viral replication		Synthesis of a single polyprotein cleaved by viral and cellular proteases to generate individual viral proteins; replication of viral genome in RCs associated to ER-derived membranes	Inferred from other Alphaviruses: synthesis of two polyproteins from two ORFs autoproteolytically cleaved to generate individual viral proteins; replication of viral genome in RCs associated to endosomes/lysosomes-derived membranes	[5,180–190]
Place of assembly		ER membrane	Plasma membrane	[191–194]
Mechanism of release		Secretion	Budding at the plasma membrane	

+: positive tropism and positive interaction with the indicated receptor. -: negative tropism and negative interaction with the indicated receptor. NI: no information available.

Table 2. Comparison of CHIKV and DENV tropism's in humans and of the replicative strategies developed by these viruses in mammalian cells.

Also, fusion of alphaviruses seems to depend on the activity of the TSPAN9 tetraspanin protein, as depletion of the protein selectively blocks the fusion of Semliki Forest Virus (SFV) without altering the one of DENV. TSPAN9 may control the correct routing of the viruses to the early endosomes and maintain these compartments in a permissive state for alphaviruses fusion but not for flaviviruses [161].

There are also differences in the mechanisms involved in CHIKV and DENV synthesis of viral proteins, genome replication and assembly of the viral components to form mature infectious virions (Table 2). In the case of CHIKV, almost all the information about these processes has been inferred from studies performed with related alphaviruses such as SFV and Sindbis Virus (SINV). Once the viral genome is released into the cytoplasm, it is translated from two different open reading frames to generate the nonstructural (nsP1234) and structural (C-pE2-6K-E1) polyproteins [5, 180]. The nonstructural polyprotein is cleaved by the nsP2 viral protease to generate the individual nonstructural proteins that are going to form replication complexes

(RCs) in charge of the viral genome replication [195]. These RCs are associated to virus-induced membranous cytoplasmic structures that are derived from the endosomes and lysosomes [181–184]. The structural polyprotein is cleaved autoproteolitically by the C protein which is released in the cytoplasm. The rest of the polyprotein (pE2-6K-E1) is translocated to the endoplasmic reticulum (ER) where it is further processed by the host cell signal peptidase to generate the individual PE2, 6K, and E1 proteins [196]. These proteins are then routed to the plasma membrane through the Golgi network where the furin-like protease cleaves the pE2 to generate the E2 and E3 mature proteins. At the plasma membrane, all the structural proteins gather together along with the genomic viral RNA, and the interaction between the C and E2 proteins drives the budding process, giving rise to enveloped virions that are released to external medium [191, 192].

In the case of flaviviruses, upon release of the viral genome into the cytoplasm, the nonstructural (NS) and structural proteins are translated from a single ORF to generate a large polyprotein that translocates to the membrane of the ER. There, the viral NS2B-NS3 protease and the host cell signalase cleave the polyprotein to generate the individual nonstructural proteins and the C, pre-Membrane (prM) and E proteins [185–188]. The nonstructural proteins form RCs associated to virus-induced membranes derived from the ER, known as vesicle packets, and drive the replication of the viral genome [189, 190]. Flavivirus assembly results from the association of C proteins with the genomic RNA into ER-derived membranes where all the structural proteins are displayed. The assembly generates immature viral particles that acquire their lipid envelope by budding into the lumen of the ER. These particles are routed through the Golgi network, and final maturation occurs at the trans-Golgi where the furin cleaves the prM to generate the mature M protein. These mature virions are then secreted to the external medium [193, 194].

Thus, the different replicative strategies, assembly compartments and release mechanisms used by flaviviruses and alphaviruses, may allow CHIKV and DENV to replicate simultaneously without a substantial overlap in their cellular requirements.

Another tempting possibility is that both viruses contribute to shut-off the antiviral cellular mechanisms, creating a favorable environment for viral replication. For example, the type I interferon response (IFN I) represents an important antiviral response against DENV and CHIKV. Accordingly, treatment with either IFN-α or IFN-β suppresses the replication of both viruses in cell culture [170, 197, 198]. Therefore, CHIKV and DENV have developed strategies to counteract the cellular defense system. In the case of DENV, almost all the nonstructural proteins are able to alter the IFN I response. Indeed, NS2A and NS4B inhibit the interferon α/β response by blocking the activation and translocation of the signal transducer and activator of transcription 1 (STAT1) to the nucleus and the subsequent transcription of antiviral genes [199]. Furthermore, DENV NS2B/NS3 proteolytic activity has been involved in the inhibition of type I IFN response by degrading human stimulator of interferon gene (STING) protein in dendritic cells, which are known to be a primary target of DENV [200, 201]. STING is an adaptor protein that senses nucleic acids of incoming pathogens and triggers signaling pathways that activate the expression of IFN I and proinflammatory cytokines [202, 203]. DENV NS5 protein is also able to interact with STAT2 and bridge the protein to cellular ubiquitin ligases, thereby promoting the STAT2 proteasome-dependent degradation [204, 205].

In the case of CHIKV, it has been established that nsP2 is a potent inhibitor of the type I and II IFN-stimulated JAK-STAT signaling by blocking the phosphorylation of STAT-1 and its translocation to the nucleus [206]. Therefore, a scenario could be envisioned in which the IFN response inhibitory effects of CHIKV and DENV nonstructural proteins are added to create a more potent shut-off of the antiviral cellular response that would be beneficial for both viruses.

5. Perspectives and challenges

Very little is known about the ecology and biology of CHIKV and DENV coinfections. Since a decade, the increasing number of reported cases in Asia, Africa, and America shows that it is a generalized phenomenon that has been underestimated. Both *Ae. aegypti* and *Ae. albopictus* mosquito vectors are able to transmit these viruses and have been directly involved in some of the coinfection cases described to the date. A particular attention has been paid to *Ae. albopictus*, as: (i) it is the only species that has been shown to sustain concomitant infection by both viruses in natural conditions: (ii) it is an aggressive species that is spreading worldwide and displacing resident populations of *Ae. aegypti*; (iii) it is installed in the northern hemisphere contrary to its *Ae. aegypti* counterpart, representing a threat for the transmission of CHIKV and DENV among nonimmune populations in Europe and North America. However, further studies are required to evaluate the precise impact of each *Aedes* species on the transmission of DENV and CHIKV taking into account that infection susceptibility, vector ecology and interactions among sympatric populations of *Aedes* mosquitoes can deeply vary between geographical regions. A better understanding of these dynamics at the local level may allow to adapt vector control measures to each situation according to the results obtained from the field.

The clinical consequences of CHIKV/DENV coinfections remain largely unknown. Indeed, the available data is not enough to conclude if the concomitant infection by both viruses is able to aggravate the clinical symptoms caused by DENV and CHIKV monoinfections. A systematic and larger clinical survey should be done to assess if coinfections are associated to severe forms of dengue and chikungunya diseases. This is particularly important, as clinical studies may justify further research on the pathogenesis of CHIKV/DENV coinfections to understand the immunological events that are triggered. This information could be useful to design and improve prophylactic vaccines against each virus.

Finally, the almost complete absence of information on the cell biology of CHIKV and DENV coinfections open a large range of research opportunities. In that sense, the mechanisms by which the viruses avoid competition or find cooperative mechanisms to replicate simultaneously are two major axes of research that should be addressed more deeply. By identifying common cellular targets of both viruses, antiviral drugs may be designed to treat coinfected patients or even to produce vaccines that are able to concomitantly immunize against both viruses.

Acknowledgements

This work was supported by grants from the Agence Nationale de la Recherche (grants ANR-12-BSV3-0004-01 and IRD.

Author details

Manuel Perera-Lecoin[1], Natthanej Luplertlop[2], Pornapat Surasombatpattana[3], Florian Liégeois[1], Rodolphe Hamel[1], Supatra Thongrungkiat[2], Ronald Enrique Morales Vargas[2], Hans Yssel[4] and Dorothée Missé[1*]

*Address all correspondence to: dorothee.misse@ird.fr

1 Laboratoire MIVEGEC, UMR 224 IRD/CNRS/UM1, Montpellier, France

2 Faculty of Tropical Medicine, Mahidol University, Bangkok, Thailand

3 Pathology Department, Prince of Songkla University, Songkla, Thailand

4 Centre d'Immunologie et des Maladies Infectieuses, Inserm, U1135, Sorbonne Universités, UPMC, APHP Hôpital Pitié-Salpêtrière, Paris, France

References

[1] Bhatt S, Gething PW, Brady OJ, Messina JP, Farlow AW, et al. (2013) The global distribution and burden of dengue. Nature 496: 504–507.

[2] Gubler DKG, Flaviviruses ML (2007). In: Knipe DM, Griffin DE, Lamb RA, Martin MA, Roizman B, editors. Fields Virology. 5th ed. Philadelphia: Lippincott Williams & Wilkins.

[3] Gubler DJ (1998) Dengue and dengue hemorrhagic fever. Clin Microbiol Rev 11: 480–496.

[4] Deen J, Lum L, Martinez E, Huat Tan L (2009) Clinical Management and Delivery of Clinical Services. Dengue Guidelines for Diagnosis, Treatment, Prevention and Control WHO Library Cataloguing-in-Publication Data.

[5] Leung JY, Ng MM, Chu JJ (2011) Replication of alphaviruses: a review on the entry process of alphaviruses into cells. Adv Virol 2011: 249640.

[6] Schwartz O, Albert ML (2010) Biology and pathogenesis of chikungunya virus. Nat Rev Microbiol 8: 491–500.

[7] Gerardin P, Barau G, Michault A, Bintner M, Randrianaivo H, et al. (2008) Multidisciplinary prospective study of mother-to-child chikungunya virus infections on the island of La Reunion. PLoS Med 5: e60.

[8] Powers AM, Logue CH (2007) Changing patterns of chikungunya virus: re-emergence of a zoonotic arbovirus. J Gen Virol 88: 2363–2377.

[9] Fischer M, Staples JE (2014) Notes from the field: chikungunya virus spreads in the Americas - Caribbean and South America, 2013-2014. MMWR Morb Mortal Wkly Rep 63: 500–501.

[10] Johansson MA, Powers AM, Pesik N, Cohen NJ, Staples JE (2014) Nowcasting the spread of chikungunya virus in the Americas. PLoS One 9: e104915.

[11] Christie J (1881) On epidemics of dengue fever: Their diffusion and etiology. Glasgow Med J 16: 161–176.

[12] Rush AB (1789) An account of the bilious remitting fever, as it appeared in Philadelphia in the summer and autumn of the year 1980. Philadelphia: Prichard and Hall.

[13] Bylon D (1780) Korte Aantekening, wegens eene Algemeene Ziekte, Doorgaans Genaamd de Knokkel Koorts. Amsterdam: Johannes Allart.

[14] Siler JF, Hall MW, Hitchens AP (1926) Dengue: Its history, epidemiology, mechanism of transmission, etiology, clinical manifestations, immunity, and prevention. Philippine J Sci 26: 1–252.

[15] Simmons JS, St John JH, Reynolds FHK (1931) Experimental studies of dengue. Philippine J Sci 44: 1–252.

[16] Sabin AB (1952) Research on dengue during World War II. Am J Trop Med Hyg 1: 30–50.

[17] Hammon WM, Sather GE (1964) Virological Findings in the 1960 Hemorrhagic Fever Epidemic (Dengue) in Thailand. Am J Trop Med Hyg 13: 629–641.

[18] Vasilakis N, Weaver SC (2008) The history and evolution of human dengue emergence. Adv Virus Res 72: 1–76.

[19] Twiddy SS, Holmes EC, Rambaut A (2003) Inferring the rate and time-scale of dengue virus evolution. Mol Biol Evol 20: 122–129.

[20] Holmes EC, Twiddy SS (2003) The origin, emergence and evolutionary genetics of dengue virus. Infect Genet Evol 3: 19–28.

[21] Weaver SC, Reisen WK (2010) Present and future arboviral threats. Antiviral Res 85: 328–345.

[22] Mackenzie JS, Gubler DJ, Petersen LR (2004) Emerging flaviviruses: the spread and resurgence of Japanese encephalitis, West Nile and dengue viruses. Nat Med 10: S98–109.

[23] Gubler DJ (2002) Epidemic dengue/dengue hemorrhagic fever as a public health, social and economic problem in the 21st century. Trends Microbiol 10: 100–103.

[24] Gubler DJ (1989) Aedes aegypti and Aedes aegypti-borne disease control in the 1990s: top down or bottom up. Charles Franklin Craig Lecture. Am J Trop Med Hyg 40: 571–578.

[25] Ponlawat A, Harrington LC (2005) Blood feeding patterns of Aedes aegypti and Aedes albopictus in Thailand. J Med Entomol 42: 844–849.

[26] Sivan A, Shriram AN, Sunish IP, Vidhya PT (2015) Host-feeding pattern of Aedes aegypti and Aedes albopictus (Diptera: Culicidae) in heterogeneous landscapes of South Andaman, Andaman and Nicobar Islands, India. Parasitol Res.

[27] Harrington LC, Edman JD, Scott TW (2001) Why do female Aedes aegypti (Diptera: Culicidae) feed preferentially and frequently on human blood? J Med Entomol 38: 411–422.

[28] Rodhain F (1996) Ecology of Aedes aegypti in Africa and Asia. Bull Soc Pathol Exot 89: 103–106.

[29] Khin MM, Than KA (1983) Transovarial transmission of dengue 2 virus by Aedes aegypti in nature. Am J Trop Med Hyg 32: 590–594.

[30] Benedict MQ, Levine RS, Hawley WA, Lounibos LP (2007) Spread of the tiger: global risk of invasion by the mosquito Aedes albopictus. Vector Borne Zoonotic Dis 7: 76–85.

[31] Vazeille M, Mousson L, Rakatoarivony I, Villeret R, Rodhain F, et al. (2001) Population genetic structure and competence as a vector for dengue type 2 virus of Aedes aegypti and Aedes albopictus from Madagascar. Am J Trop Med Hyg 65: 491–497.

[32] Rosen L, Roseboom LE, Gubler DJ, Lien JC, Chaniotis BN (1985) Comparative susceptibility of mosquito species and strains to oral and parenteral infection with dengue and Japanese encephalitis viruses. Am J Trop Med Hyg 34: 603–615.

[33] Alto BW, Reiskind MH, Lounibos LP (2008) Size alters susceptibility of vectors to dengue virus infection and dissemination. Am J Trop Med Hyg 79: 688–695.

[34] Jumali, Sunarto, Gubler DJ, Nalim S, Eram S, et al. (1979) Epidemic dengue hemorrhagic fever in rural Indonesia. III. Entomological studies. Am J Trop Med Hyg 28: 717–724.

[35] Whitehead RH, Yuill TM, Gould DJ, Simasathien P (1971) Experimental infection of Aedes aegypti and Aedes albopictus with dengue viruses. Trans R Soc Trop Med Hyg 65: 661–667.

[36] Moncayo AC, Fernandez Z, Ortiz D, Diallo M, Sall A, et al. (2004) Dengue emergence and adaptation to peridomestic mosquitoes. Emerg Infect Dis 10: 1790–1796.

[37] Richards SL, Anderson SL, Alto BW (2012) Vector competence of Aedes aegypti and Aedes albopictus (Diptera: Culicidae) for dengue virus in the Florida Keys. J Med Entomol 49: 942–946.

[38] Lambrechts L, Scott TW, Gubler DJ (2010) Consequences of the expanding global distribution of Aedes albopictus for dengue virus transmission. PLoS Negl Trop Dis 4: e646.

[39] Failloux AB, Vazeille M, Rodhain F (2002) Geographic genetic variation in populations of the dengue virus vector Aedes aegypti. J Mol Evol 55: 653–663.

[40] Armstrong PM, Rico-Hesse R (2003) Efficiency of dengue serotype 2 virus strains to infect and disseminate in Aedes aegypti. Am J Trop Med Hyg 68: 539–544.

[41] Armstrong PM, Rico-Hesse R (2001) Differential susceptibility of Aedes aegypti to infection by the American and Southeast Asian genotypes of dengue type 2 virus. Vector Borne Zoonotic Dis 1: 159–168.

[42] Almeida AP, Baptista SS, Sousa CA, Novo MT, Ramos HC, et al. (2005) Bioecology and vectorial capacity of Aedes albopictus (Diptera: Culicidae) in Macao, China, in relation to dengue virus transmission. J Med Entomol 42: 419–428.

[43] Effler PV, Pang L, Kitsutani P, Vorndam V, Nakata M, et al. (2005) Dengue fever, Hawaii, 2001-2002. Emerg Infect Dis 11: 742–749.

[44] Pierre V, Thiria J, Rachou E, Sissoko D, Lassalle C, et al. (2005) Epidémie de dengue 1 à la Réunion en 2004. Journal de Veille Sanitaire.

[45] Ramchurn SK, Moheeput K, Goorah SS (2009) An analysis of a short-lived outbreak of dengue fever in Mauritius. Euro Surveill 14.

[46] La Ruche G, Souares Y, Armengaud A, Peloux-Petiot F, Delaunay P, et al. (2010) First two autochthonous dengue virus infections in metropolitan France, September 2010. Euro Surveill 15: 19676.

[47] Gjenero-Margan I, Aleraj B, Krajcar D, Lesnikar V, Klobucar A, et al. (2011) Autochthonous dengue fever in Croatia, August-September 2010. Euro Surveill 16.

[48] Medlock JM, Hansford KM, Schaffner F, Versteirt V, Hendrickx G, et al. (2012) A review of the invasive mosquitoes in Europe: ecology, public health risks, and control options. Vector Borne Zoonotic Dis 12: 435–447.

[49] Hawley WA, Reiter P, Copeland RS, Pumpuni CB, Craig GB, Jr. (1987) Aedes albopictus in North America: probable introduction in used tires from northern Asia. Science 236: 1114–1116.

[50] Delatte H, Gimonneau G, Triboire A, Fontenille D (2009) Influence of temperature on immature development, survival, longevity, fecundity, and gonotrophic cycles of Aedes albopictus, vector of chikungunya and dengue in the Indian Ocean. J Med Entomol 46: 33–41.

[51] Hanson SM, Craig GB, Jr. (1995) Aedes albopictus (Diptera: Culicidae) eggs: field survivorship during northern Indiana winters. J Med Entomol 32: 599–604.

[52] Hanson SM, Craig GB, Jr. (1995) Relationship between cold hardiness and supercooling point in Aedes albopictus eggs. J Am Mosq Control Assoc 11: 35–38.

[53] Briegel H, Timmermann SE (2001) Aedes albopictus (Diptera: Culicidae): physiological aspects of development and reproduction. J Med Entomol 38: 566–571.

[54] Paupy C, Delatte H, Bagny L, Corbel V, Fontenille D (2009) Aedes albopictus, an arbovirus vector: from the darkness to the light. Microbes Infect 11: 1177–1185.

[55] Kamgang B, Nchoutpouen E, Simard F, Paupy C (2012) Notes on the blood-feeding behavior of Aedes albopictus (Diptera: Culicidae) in Cameroon. Parasit Vectors 5: 57.

[56] Richards SL, Ponnusamy L, Unnasch TR, Hassan HK, Apperson CS (2006) Host-feeding patterns of Aedes albopictus (Diptera: Culicidae) in relation to availability of human and domestic animals in suburban landscapes of central North Carolina. J Med Entomol 43: 543–551.

[57] Delatte H, Desvars A, Bouetard A, Bord S, Gimonneau G, et al. (2010) Blood-feeding behavior of Aedes albopictus, a vector of Chikungunya on La Reunion. Vector Borne Zoonotic Dis 10: 249–258.

[58] Raharimalala FN, Ravaomanarivo LH, Ravelonandro P, Rafarasoa LS, Zouache K, et al. (2012) Biogeography of the two major arbovirus mosquito vectors, Aedes aegypti and Aedes albopictus (Diptera, Culicidae), in Madagascar. Parasit Vectors 5: 56.

[59] Simard F, Nchoutpouen E, Toto JC, Fontenille D (2005) Geographic distribution and breeding site preference of Aedes albopictus and Aedes aegypti (Diptera: culicidae) in Cameroon, Central Africa. J Med Entomol 42: 726–731.

[60] Juliano SA, Lounibos LP, O'Meara GF (2004) A field test for competitive effects of Aedes albopictus on A. aegypti in South Florida: differences between sites of coexistence and exclusion? Oecologia 139: 583–593.

[61] Braks MA, Honorio NA, Lourencqo-De-Oliveira R, Juliano SA, Lounibos LP (2003) Convergent habitat segregation of Aedes aegypti and Aedes albopictus (Diptera: Culicidae) in southeastern Brazil and Florida. J Med Entomol 40: 785–794.

[62] Daugherty MP, Alto BW, Juliano SA (2000) Invertebrate carcasses as a resource for competing Aedes albopictus and Aedes aegypti (Diptera: Culicidae). J Med Entomol 37: 364–372.

[63] Braks MAH, Honório NA, Lounibos LP, Lourenço-De-Oliveira R, Juliano SA (2004) Interspecific Competition Between Two Invasive Species of Container Mosquitoes, Aedes aegypti and Aedes albopictus (Diptera: Culicidae), in Brazil. 130–139 p.

[64] Lumsden WH (1955) An epidemic of virus disease in Southern Province, Tanganyika Territory, in 1952-53. II. General description and epidemiology. Trans R Soc Trop Med Hyg 49: 33–57.

[65] Ross RW (1956) The Newala epidemic. III. The virus: isolation, pathogenic properties and relationship to the epidemic. J Hyg (Lond) 54: 177–191.

[66] Weaver SC, Forrester NL (2015) Chikungunya: Evolutionary history and recent epidemic spread. Antiviral Res 120: 32–39.

[67] Carey DE (1971) Chikungunya and dengue: a case of mistaken identity? J Hist Med Allied Sci 26: 243–262.

[68] Halstead SB (2015) Reappearance of chikungunya, formerly called dengue, in the Americas. Emerg Infect Dis 21: 557–561.

[69] Volk SM, Chen R, Tsetsarkin KA, Adams AP, Garcia TI, et al. (2010) Genome-scale phylogenetic analyses of chikungunya virus reveal independent emergences of recent epidemics and various evolutionary rates. J Virol 84: 6497–6504.

[70] Weinbren MP, Haddow AJ, Williams MC (1958) The occurrence of Chikungunya virus in Uganda. I. Isolation from mosquitoes. Trans R Soc Trop Med Hyg 52: 253–257.

[71] Jupp PG, McIntosh BM (1990) Aedes furcifer and other mosquitoes as vectors of chikungunya virus at Mica, northeastern Transvaal, South Africa. J Am Mosq Control Assoc 6: 415–420.

[72] McCarthy MC, Haberberger RL, Salib AW, Soliman BA, El-Tigani A, et al. (1996) Evaluation of arthropod-borne viruses and other infectious disease pathogens as the causes of febrile illnesses in the Khartoum Province of Sudan. J Med Virol 48: 141–146.

[73] Thonnon J, Spiegel A, Diallo M, Diallo A, Fontenille D (1999) Chikungunya virus outbreak in Senegal in 1996 and 1997. Bull Soc Pathol Exot 92: 79–82.

[74] Peyrefitte CN, Rousset D, Pastorino BA, Pouillot R, Bessaud M, et al. (2007) Chikungunya virus, Cameroon, 2006. Emerg Infect Dis 13: 768–771.

[75] Peyrefitte CN, Bessaud M, Pastorino BA, Gravier P, Plumet S, et al. (2008) Circulation of Chikungunya virus in Gabon, 2006-2007. J Med Virol 80: 430–433.

[76] Mombouli JV, Bitsindou P, Elion DO, Grolla A, Feldmann H, et al. (2013) Chikungunya virus infection, Brazzaville, Republic of Congo, 2011. Emerg Infect Dis 19: 1542–1543.

[77] Hammon WM, Rudnick A, Sather GE (1960) Viruses associated with epidemic hemorrhagic fevers of the Philippines and Thailand. Science 131: 1102–1103.

[78] Pavri KM (1964) Presence of Chikungunya Antibodies in Human Sera Collected from Calcutta and Jamshedpur before 1963. Indian J Med Res 52: 698–702.

[79] Hermon YE (1967) Virological investigations of Arbovirus infections in Ceylon, with special reference to the recent Chikungunya fever epidemic. Ceylon Med J 12: 81–92.

[80] Lahariya C, Pradhan SK (2006) Emergence of chikungunya virus in Indian subcontinent after 32 years: A review. J Vector Borne Dis 43: 151–160.

[81] Yergolkar PN, Tandale BV, Arankalle VA, Sathe PS, Sudeep AB, et al. (2006) Chikungunya outbreaks caused by African genotype, India. Emerg Infect Dis 12: 1580–1583.

[82] Kularatne SA, Gihan MC, Weerasinghe SC, Gunasena S (2009) Concurrent outbreaks of Chikungunya and Dengue fever in Kandy, Sri Lanka, 2006-07: a comparative analysis of clinical and laboratory features. Postgrad Med J 85: 342–346.

[83] Kariuki Njenga M, Nderitu L, Ledermann JP, Ndirangu A, Logue CH, et al. (2008) Tracking epidemic Chikungunya virus into the Indian Ocean from East Africa. J Gen Virol 89: 2754–2760.

[84] Chastel C (2005) [Chikungunya virus: its recent spread to the southern Indian Ocean and Reunion Island (2005-2006)]. Bull Acad Natl Med 189: 1827–1835.

[85] Higgs S (2006) The 2005-2006 Chikungunya epidemic in the Indian Ocean. Vector Borne Zoonotic Dis 6: 115–116.

[86] Bonn D (2006) How did chikungunya reach the Indian Ocean? Lancet Infect Dis 6: 543.

[87] Josseran L, Paquet C, Zehgnoun A, Caillere N, Le Tertre A, et al. (2006) Chikungunya disease outbreak, Reunion Island. Emerg Infect Dis 12: 1994–1995.

[88] Sam IC, Chan YF, Chan SY, Loong SK, Chin HK, et al. (2009) Chikungunya virus of Asian and Central/East African genotypes in Malaysia. J Clin Virol 46: 180–183.

[89] Ng KW, Chow A, Win MK, Dimatatac F, Neo HY, et al. (2009) Clinical features and epidemiology of chikungunya infection in Singapore. Singapore Med J 50: 785–790.

[90] Theamboonlers A, Rianthavorn P, Praianantathavorn K, Wuttirattanakowit N, Poovorawan Y (2009) Clinical and molecular characterization of chikungunya virus in South Thailand. Jpn J Infect Dis 62: 303–305.

[91] Wu D, Wu J, Zhang Q, Zhong H, Ke C, et al. (2012) Chikungunya outbreak in Guangdong Province, China, 2010. Emerg Infect Dis 18: 493–495.

[92] Duong V, Andries AC, Ngan C, Sok T, Richner B, et al. (2012) Reemergence of Chikungunya virus in Cambodia. Emerg Infect Dis 18: 2066–2069.

[93] Wangchuk S, Chinnawirotpisan P, Dorji T, Tobgay T, Yoon IK, et al. (2013) Chikungunya fever outbreak, Bhutan, 2012. Emerg Infect Dis 19: 1681–1684.

[94] Organization PAHO-WH (2014) Factsheet Chikungunya.

[95] Rezza G, Nicoletti L, Angelini R, Romi R, Finarelli AC, et al. (2007) Infection with chikungunya virus in Italy: an outbreak in a temperate region. Lancet 370: 1840–1846.

[96] Grandadam M, Caro V, Plumet S, Thiberge JM, Souares Y, et al. (2011) Chikungunya virus, southeastern France. Emerg Infect Dis 17: 910–913.

[97] Paty MC, Six C, Charlet F, Heuze G, Cochet A, et al. (2014) Large number of imported chikungunya cases in mainland France, 2014: a challenge for surveillance and response. Euro Surveill 19: 20856.

[98] Leparc-Goffart I, Nougairede A, Cassadou S, Prat C, de Lamballerie X (2014) Chikungunya in the Americas. Lancet 383: 514.

[99] Organization PHO-WH (2016) Chikungunya- PAHO/WHO Data, Maps and Statistics. Panamerican Health Organization Website.

[100] Kosasih H, de Mast Q, Widjaja S, Sudjana P, Antonjaya U, et al. (2013) Evidence for endemic chikungunya virus infections in Bandung, Indonesia. PLoS Negl Trop Dis 7: e2483.

[101] Tan KK, Sy AK, Tandoc AO, Khoo JJ, Sulaiman S, et al. (2015) Independent Emergence of the Cosmopolitan Asian Chikungunya Virus, Philippines 2012. Sci Rep 5: 12279.

[102] Nhan TX, Musso D (2015) The burden of chikungunya in the Pacific. Clin Microbiol Infect 21: e47–48.

[103] Coffey LL, Failloux AB, Weaver SC (2014) Chikungunya virus-vector interactions. Viruses 6: 4628–4663.

[104] Schuffenecker I, Iteman I, Michault A, Murri S, Frangeul L, et al. (2006) Genome microevolution of chikungunya viruses causing the Indian Ocean outbreak. PLoS Med 3: e263.

[105] Tsetsarkin KA, Vanlandingham DL, McGee CE, Higgs S (2007) A single mutation in chikungunya virus affects vector specificity and epidemic potential. PLoS Pathog 3: e201.

[106] Vazeille M, Moutailler S, Coudrier D, Rousseaux C, Khun H, et al. (2007) Two Chikungunya isolates from the outbreak of La Reunion (Indian Ocean) exhibit different patterns of infection in the mosquito, Aedes albopictus. PLoS One 2: e1168.

[107] de Lamballerie X, Leroy E, Charrel RN, Ttsetsarkin K, Higgs S, et al. (2008) Chikungunya virus adapts to tiger mosquito via evolutionary convergence: a sign of things to come? Virol J 5: 33.

[108] Tsetsarkin KA, McGee CE, Higgs S (2011) Chikungunya virus adaptation to Aedes albopictus mosquitoes does not correlate with acquisition of cholesterol dependence or decreased pH threshold for fusion reaction. Virol J 8: 376.

[109] Niyas KP, Abraham R, Unnikrishnan RN, Mathew T, Nair S, et al. (2010) Molecular characterization of Chikungunya virus isolates from clinical samples and adult Aedes albopictus mosquitoes emerged from larvae from Kerala, South India. Virol J 7: 189.

[110] Tsetsarkin KA, Weaver SC (2011) Sequential adaptive mutations enhance efficient vector switching by Chikungunya virus and its epidemic emergence. PLoS Pathog 7: e1002412.

[111] Tsetsarkin KA, Chen R, Leal G, Forrester N, Higgs S, et al. (2011) Chikungunya virus emergence is constrained in Asia by lineage-specific adaptive landscapes. Proc Natl Acad Sci U S A 108: 7872–7877.

[112] Stapleford KA, Coffey LL, Lay S, Borderia AV, Duong V, et al. (2014) Emergence and transmission of arbovirus evolutionary intermediates with epidemic potential. Cell Host Microbe 15: 706–716.

[113] Whitehead SS, Blaney JE, Durbin AP, Murphy BR (2007) Prospects for a dengue virus vaccine. Nat Rev Microbiol 5: 518–528.

[114] Vasilakis N, Cardosa J, Hanley KA, Holmes EC, Weaver SC (2011) Fever from the forest: prospects for the continued emergence of sylvatic dengue virus and its impact on public health. Nat Rev Microbiol 9: 532–541.

[115] Tsetsarkin KA, Chen R, Sherman MB, Weaver SC (2011) Chikungunya virus: evolution and genetic determinants of emergence. Curr Opin Virol 1: 310–317.

[116] Myers RM, Carey DE (1967) Concurrent isolation from patient of two arboviruses, Chikungunya and dengue type 2. Science 157: 1307–1308.

[117] Carey DE, Myers RM, DeRanitz CM, Jadhav M, Reuben R (1969) The 1964 chikungunya epidemic at Vellore, South India, including observations on concurrent dengue. Trans R Soc Trop Med Hyg 63: 434–445.

[118] Halstead SB, Nimmannitya S, Margiotta MR (1969) Dengue d chikungunya virus infection in man in Thailand, 1962-1964. II. Observations on disease in outpatients. Am J Trop Med Hyg 18: 972–983.

[119] Schilling S, Emmerich P, Gunther S, Schmidt-Chanasit J (2009) Dengue and Chikungunya virus co-infection in a German traveller. J Clin Virol 45: 163–164.

[120] Parreira R, Centeno-Lima S, Lopes A, Portugal-Calisto D, Constantino A, et al. (2014) Dengue virus serotype 4 and chikungunya virus coinfection in a traveller returning from Luanda, Angola, January 2014. Euro Surveill 19.

[121] (2006) Outbreak news. Chikungunya and dengue, south-west Indian Ocean. Wkly Epidemiol Rec 81: 106–108.

[122] Nayar SK, Noridah O, Paranthaman V, Ranjit K, Norizah I, et al. (2007) Co-infection of dengue virus and chikungunya virus in two patients with acute febrile illness. Med J Malaysia 62: 335–336.

[123] Ratsitorahina M, Harisoa J, Ratovonjato J, Biacabe S, Reynes JM, et al. (2008) Outbreak of dengue and Chikungunya fevers, Toamasina, Madagascar, 2006. Emerg Infect Dis 14: 1135–1137.

[124] Caron M, Paupy C, Grard G, Becquart P, Mombo I, et al. (2012) Recent introduction and rapid dissemination of Chikungunya virus and Dengue virus serotype 2 associated with human and mosquito coinfections in Gabon, central Africa. Clin Infect Dis 55: e45–53.

[125] Leroy EM, Nkoghe D, Ollomo B, Nze-Nkogue C, Becquart P, et al. (2009) Concurrent chikungunya and dengue virus infections during simultaneous outbreaks, Gabon, 2007. Emerg Infect Dis 15: 591–593.

[126] Baba M, Logue CH, Oderinde B, Abdulmaleek H, Williams J, et al. (2013) Evidence of arbovirus co-infection in suspected febrile malaria and typhoid patients in Nigeria. J Infect Dev Ctries 7: 51–59.

[127] Chahar HS, Bharaj P, Dar L, Guleria R, Kabra SK, et al. (2009) Co-infections with chikungunya virus and dengue virus in Delhi, India. Emerg Infect Dis 15: 1077–1080.

[128] Chang SF, Su CL, Shu PY, Yang CF, Liao TL, et al. (2010) Concurrent isolation of chikungunya virus and dengue virus from a patient with coinfection resulting from a trip to Singapore. J Clin Microbiol 48: 4586–4589.

[129] Saswat T, Kumar A, Kumar S, Mamidi P, Muduli S, et al. (2015) High rates of co-infection of Dengue and Chikungunya virus in Odisha and Maharashtra, India during 2013. Infect Genet Evol 35: 134–141.

[130] Omarjee R, Prat C, Flusin O, Boucau S, Tenebray B, et al. (2014) Importance of case definition to monitor ongoing outbreak of chikungunya virus on a background of actively circulating dengue virus, St Martin, December 2013 to January 2014. Euro Surveill 19.

[131] Raut CG, Rao NM, Sinha DP, Hanumaiah H, Manjunatha MJ (2015) Chikungunya, dengue, and malaria co-infection after travel to Nigeria, India. Emerg Infect Dis 21: 907–909.

[132] Kalawat U, Sharma KK, Reddy SG (2011) Prevalence of dengue and chickungunya fever and their co-infection. Indian J Pathol Microbiol 54: 844–846.

[133] Moyen N, Thiberville SD, Pastorino B, Nougairede A, Thirion L, et al. (2014) First reported chikungunya fever outbreak in the republic of Congo, 2011. PLoS One 9: e115938.

[134] Kraemer MU, Sinka ME, Duda KA, Mylne A, Shearer FM, et al. (2015) The global compendium of Aedes aegypti and Ae. albopictus occurrence. Sci Data 2: 150035.

[135] Paupy C, Ollomo B, Kamgang B, Moutailler S, Rousset D, et al. (2010) Comparative role of Aedes albopictus and Aedes aegypti in the emergence of Dengue and Chikungunya in central Africa. Vector Borne Zoonotic Dis 10: 259–266.

[136] Coffinet T, Mourou JR, Pradines B, Toto JC, Jarjaval F, et al. (2007) First record of Aedes albopictus in Gabon. J Am Mosq Control Assoc 23: 471–472.

[137] Krueger A, Hagen RM (2007) Short communication: first record of Aedes albopictus in Gabon, Central Africa. Trop Med Int Health 12: 1105–1107.

[138] Vazeille M, Mousson L, Martin E, Failloux AB (2010) Orally co-Infected Aedes albopictus from La Reunion Island, Indian Ocean, can deliver both dengue and chikungunya infectious viral particles in their saliva. PLoS Negl Trop Dis 4: e706.

[139] Rohani A, Potiwat R, Zamree I, Lee HL (2009) Refractoriness of Aedes aegypti (Linnaeus) to dual infection with dengue and chikungunya virus. Southeast Asian J Trop Med Public Health 40: 443–448.

[140] Rico-Hesse R (2003) Microevolution and virulence of dengue viruses. Adv Virus Res 59: 315–341.

[141] Guzman MG, Kouri GP, Bravo J, Soler M, Vazquez S, et al. (1990) Dengue hemorrhagic fever in Cuba, 1981: a retrospective seroepidemiologic study. Am J Trop Med Hyg 42: 179–184.

[142] de la CSB, Garcia G, Perez AB, Morier L, Alvarez M, et al. (2006) Ethnicity and difference in dengue virus-specific memory T cell responses in Cuban individuals. Viral Immunol 19: 662–668.

[143] Figueiredo MA, Rodrigues LC, Barreto ML, Lima JW, Costa MC, et al. (2010) Allergies and diabetes as risk factors for dengue hemorrhagic fever: results of a case control study. PLoS Negl Trop Dis 4: e699.

[144] Kliks SC, Nisalak A, Brandt WE, Wahl L, Burke DS (1989) Antibody-dependent enhancement of dengue virus growth in human monocytes as a risk factor for dengue hemorrhagic fever. Am J Trop Med Hyg 40: 444–451.

[145] Halstead SB (1988) Pathogenesis of dengue: challenges to molecular biology. Science 239: 476–481.

[146] Vaughn DW, Green S, Kalayanarooj S, Innis BL, Nimmannitya S, et al. (2000) Dengue viremia titer, antibody response pattern, and virus serotype correlate with disease severity. J Infect Dis 181: 2–9.

[147] Libraty DH, Young PR, Pickering D, Endy TP, Kalayanarooj S, et al. (2002) High circulating levels of the dengue virus nonstructural protein xlink early in dengue illness

correlate with the development of dengue hemorrhagic fever. J Infect Dis 186: 1165–1168.

[148] Anderson R, Wang S, Osiowy C, Issekutz AC (1997) Activation of endothelial cells via antibody-enhanced dengue virus infection of peripheral blood monocytes. J Virol 71: 4226–4232.

[149] Chaturvedi UC, Agarwal R, Elbishbishi EA, Mustafa AS (2000) Cytokine cascade in dengue hemorrhagic fever: implications for pathogenesis. FEMS Immunol Med Microbiol 28: 183–188.

[150] Chareonsirisuthigul T, Kalayanarooj S, Ubol S (2007) Dengue virus (DENV) antibody-dependent enhancement of infection upregulates the production of anti-inflammatory cytokines, but suppresses anti-DENV free radical and pro-inflammatory cytokine production, in THP-1 cells. J Gen Virol 88: 365–375.

[151] Fazekas de St G, Webster RG (1966) Disquisitions of Original Antigenic Sin. I. Evidence in man. J Exp Med 124: 331–345.

[152] Mongkolsapaya J, Duangchinda T, Dejnirattisai W, Vasanawathana S, Avirutnan P, et al. (2006) T cell responses in dengue hemorrhagic fever: are cross-reactive T cells suboptimal? J Immunol 176: 3821–3829.

[153] Nkoghe D, Kassa RF, Bisvigou U, Caron M, Grard G, et al. (2012) No clinical or biological difference between Chikungunya and Dengue Fever during the 2010 Gabonese outbreak. Infect Dis Rep 4: e5.

[154] Tchankouo-Nguetcheu S, Khun H, Pincet L, Roux P, Bahut M, et al. (2010) Differential protein modulation in midguts of Aedes aegypti infected with chikungunya and dengue 2 viruses. PLoS One 5.

[155] Potiwat R, Komalamisra N, Thavara U, Tawatsin A, Siriyasatien P (2011) Competitive suppression between chikungunya and dengue virus in Aedes albopictus c6/36 cell line. Southeast Asian J Trop Med Public Health 42: 1388–1394.

[156] Nuckols JT, Huang YJ, Higgs S, Miller AL, Pyles RB, et al. (2015) Evaluation of Simultaneous Transmission of Chikungunya Virus and Dengue Virus Type 2 in Infected Aedes aegypti and Aedes albopictus (Diptera: Culicidae). J Med Entomol 52: 447–451.

[157] Wintachai P, Wikan N, Kuadkitkan A, Jaimipuk T, Ubol S, et al. (2012) Identification of prohibitin as a Chikungunya virus receptor protein. J Med Virol 84: 1757–1770.

[158] Salas-Benito J, Reyes-Del Valle J, Salas-Benito M, Ceballos-Olvera I, Mosso C, et al. (2007) Evidence that the 45-kD glycoprotein, part of a putative dengue virus receptor complex in the mosquito cell line C6/36, is a heat-shock related protein. Am J Trop Med Hyg 77: 283–290.

[159] Kuadkitkan A, Wikan N, Fongsaran C, Smith DR (2010) Identification and characterization of prohibitin as a receptor protein mediating DENV-2 entry into insect cells. Virology 406: 149–161.

[160] Apte-Deshpande AD, Paingankar MS, Gokhale MD, Deobagkar DN (2014) Serratia odorifera mediated enhancement in susceptibility of Aedes aegypti for chikungunya virus. Indian J Med Res 139: 762–768.

[161] Ooi YS, Stiles KM, Liu CY, Taylor GM, Kielian M (2013) Genome-wide RNAi screen identifies novel host proteins required for alphavirus entry. PLoS Pathog 9: e1003835.

[162] Bernard E, Solignat M, Gay B, Chazal N, Higgs S, et al. (2010) Endocytosis of chikungunya virus into mammalian cells: role of clathrin and early endosomal compartments. PLoS One 5: e11479.

[163] Acosta EG, Castilla V, Damonte EB (2012) Differential requirements in endocytic trafficking for penetration of dengue virus. PLoS One 7: e44835.

[164] van der Schaar HM, Rust MJ, Chen C, van der Ende-Metselaar H, Wilschut J, et al. (2008) Dissecting the cell entry pathway of dengue virus by single-particle tracking in living cells. PLoS Pathog 4: e1000244.

[165] Zaitseva E, Yang ST, Melikov K, Pourmal S, Chernomordik LV (2010) Dengue virus ensures its fusion in late endosomes using compartment-specific lipids. PLoS Pathog 6: e1001131.

[166] Limon-Flores AY, Perez-Tapia M, Estrada-Garcia I, Vaughan G, Escobar-Gutierrez A, et al. (2005) Dengue virus inoculation to human skin explants: an effective approach to assess in situ the early infection and the effects on cutaneous dendritic cells. Int J Exp Pathol 86: 323–334.

[167] Wu SJ, Grouard-Vogel G, Sun W, Mascola JR, Brachtel E, et al. (2000) Human skin Langerhans cells are targets of dengue virus infection. Nat Med 6: 816-820.

[168] Marovich M, Grouard-Vogel G, Louder M, Eller M, Sun W, et al. (2001) Human dendritic cells as targets of dengue virus infection. J Investig Dermatol Symp Proc 6: 219–224.

[169] Bustos-Arriaga J, Garcia-Machorro J, Leon-Juarez M, Garcia-Cordero J, Santos-Argumedo L, et al. (2011) Activation of the innate immune response against DENV in normal non-transformed human fibroblasts. PLoS Negl Trop Dis 5: e1420.

[170] Sourisseau M, Schilte C, Casartelli N, Trouillet C, Guivel-Benhassine F, et al. (2007) Characterization of reemerging chikungunya virus. PLoS Pathog 3: e89.

[171] Surasombatpattana P, Hamel R, Patramool S, Luplertlop N, Thomas F, et al. (2011) Dengue virus replication in infected human keratinocytes leads to activation of antiviral innate immune responses. Infect Genet Evol 11: 1664–1673.

[172] Bernard E, Hamel R, Neyret A, Ekchariyawat P, Moles JP, et al. (2015) Human keratinocytes restrict chikungunya virus replication at a post-fusion step. Virology 476: 1–10.

[173] Perera-Lecoin M, Meertens L, Carnec X, Amara A (2014) Flavivirus entry receptors: an update. Viruses 6: 69–88.

[174] van Duijl-Richter MK, Hoornweg TE, Rodenhuis-Zybert IA, Smit JM (2015) Early Events in Chikungunya Virus Infection-From Virus CellBinding to Membrane Fusion. Viruses 7: 3647–3674.

[175] Suksanpaisan L, Susantad T, Smith DR (2009) Characterization of dengue virus entry into HepG2 cells. J Biomed Sci 16: 17.

[176] Mosso C, Galvan-Mendoza IJ, Ludert JE, del Angel RM (2008) Endocytic pathway followed by dengue virus to infect the mosquito cell line C6/36 HT. Virology 378: 193–199.

[177] Acosta EG, Castilla V, Damonte EB (2008) Functional entry of dengue virus into Aedes albopictus mosquito cells is dependent on clathrin-mediated endocytosis. J Gen Virol 89: 474–484.

[178] Peng T, Wang JL, Chen W, Zhang JL, Gao N, et al. (2009) Entry of dengue virus serotype 2 into ECV304 cells depends on clathrin-dependent endocytosis, but not on caveolae-dependent endocytosis. Can J Microbiol 55: 139–145.

[179] Solignat M, Gay B, Higgs S, Briant L, Devaux C (2009) Replication cycle of chikungunya: a re-emerging arbovirus. Virology 393: 183–197.

[180] Glanville N, Ranki M, Morser J, Kaariainen L, Smith AE (1976) Initiation of translation directed by 42S and 26S RNAs from Semliki Forest virus in vitro. Proc Natl Acad Sci U S A 73: 3059–3063.

[181] Froshauer S, Kartenbeck J, Helenius A (1988) Alphavirus RNA replicase is located on the cytoplasmic surface of endosomes and lysosomes. J Cell Biol 107: 2075–2086.

[182] Kujala P, Ikaheimonen A, Ehsani N, Vihinen H, Auvinen P, et al. (2001) Biogenesis of the Semliki Forest virus RNA replication complex. J Virol 75: 3873–3884.

[183] Salonen A, Vasiljeva L, Merits A, Magden J, Jokitalo E, et al. (2003) Properly folded nonstructural polyprotein directs the semliki forest virus replication complex to the endosomal compartment. J Virol 77: 1691–1702.

[184] Grimley PM, Berezesky IK, Friedman RM (1968) Cytoplasmic structures associated with an arbovirus infection: loci of viral ribonucleic acid synthesis. J Virol 2: 1326–1338.

[185] Amberg SM, Nestorowicz A, McCourt DW, Rice CM (1994) NS2B-3 proteinase-mediated processing in the yellow fever virus structural region: in vitro and in vivo studies. J Virol 68: 3794–3802.

[186] Yamshchikov VF, Compans RW (1994) Processing of the intracellular form of the west Nile virus capsid protein by the viral NS2B-NS3 protease: an in vitro study. J Virol 68: 5765–5771.

[187] Bartenschlager R, Miller S (2008) Molecular aspects of Dengue virus replication. Future Microbiol 3: 155–165.

[188] Stocks CE, Lobigs M (1998) Signal peptidase cleavage at the flavivirus C-prM junction: dependence on the viral NS2B-3 protease for efficient processing requires determinants in C, the signal peptide, and prM. J Virol 72: 2141–2149.

[189] Gillespie LK, Hoenen A, Morgan G, Mackenzie JM (2010) The endoplasmic reticulum provides the membrane platform for biogenesis of the flavivirus replication complex. J Virol 84: 10438–10447.

[190] Westaway EG, Mackenzie JM, Kenney MT, Jones MK, Khromykh AA (1997) Ultrastructure of Kunjin virus-infected cells: colocalization of xlink and NS3 with double-stranded RNA, and of NS2B with NS3, in virus-induced membrane structures. J Virol 71: 6650–6661.

[191] Owen KE, Kuhn RJ (1997) Alphavirus budding is dependent on the interaction between the nucleocapsid and hydrophobic amino acids on the cytoplasmic domain of the E2 envelope glycoprotein. Virology 230: 187–196.

[192] Vogel RH, Provencher SW, von Bonsdorff CH, Adrian M, Dubochet J (1986) Envelope structure of Semliki Forest virus reconstructed from cryo-electron micrographs. Nature 320: 533–535.

[193] Li L, Lok SM, Yu IM, Zhang Y, Kuhn RJ, et al. (2008) The flavivirus precursor membrane-envelope protein complex: structure and maturation. Science 319: 1830–1834.

[194] Mackenzie JM, Westaway EG (2001) Assembly and maturation of the flavivirus Kunjin virus appear to occur in the rough endoplasmic reticulum and along the secretory pathway, respectively. J Virol 75: 10787–10799.

[195] Hardy WR, Strauss JH (1989) Processing the nonstructural polyproteins of sindbis virus: nonstructural proteinase is in the C-terminal half of nsP2 and functions both in cis and in trans. J Virol 63: 4653–4664.

[196] Lobigs M, Zhao HX, Garoff H (1990) Function of Semliki Forest virus E3 peptide in virus assembly: replacement of E3 with an artificial signal peptide abolishes spike heterodimerization and surface expression of E1. J Virol 64: 4346–4355.

[197] Diamond MS, Roberts TG, Edgil D, Lu B, Ernst J, et al. (2000) Modulation of Dengue virus infection in human cells by alpha, beta, and gamma interferons. J Virol 74: 4957–4966.

[198] Schilte C, Couderc T, Chretien F, Sourisseau M, Gangneux N, et al. (2010) Type I IFN controls chikungunya virus via its action on nonhematopoietic cells. J Exp Med 207: 429–442.

[199] Munoz-Jordan JL, Sanchez-Burgos GG, Laurent-Rolle M, Garcia-Sastre A (2003) Inhibition of interferon signaling by dengue virus. Proc Natl Acad Sci U S A 100: 14333–14338.

[200] Rodriguez-Madoz JR, Belicha-Villanueva A, Bernal-Rubio D, Ashour J, Ayllon J, et al. (2010) Inhibition of the type I interferon response in human dendritic cells by dengue virus infection requires a catalytically active NS2B3 complex. J Virol 84: 9760–9774.

[201] Aguirre S, Maestre AM, Pagni S, Patel JR, Savage T, et al. (2012) DENV inhibits type I IFN production in infected cells by cleaving human STING. PLoS Pathog 8: e1002934.

[202] Barber GN (2011) STING-dependent signaling. Nat Immunol 12: 929–930.

[203] Zhang Z, Yuan B, Bao M, Lu N, Kim T, et al. (2011) The helicase DDX41 senses intracellular DNA mediated by the adaptor STING in dendritic cells. Nat Immunol 12: 959–965.

[204] Ashour J, Laurent-Rolle M, Shi PY, Garcia-Sastre A (2009) NS5 of dengue virus mediates STAT2 binding and degradation. J Virol 83: 5408–5418.

[205] Morrison J, Laurent-Rolle M, Maestre AM, Rajsbaum R, Pisanelli G, et al. (2013) Dengue virus co-opts UBR4 to degrade STAT2 and antagonize type I interferon signaling. PLoS Pathog 9: e1003265.

[206] Fros JJ, Liu WJ, Prow NA, Geertsema C, Ligtenberg M, et al. (2010) Chikungunya virus nonstructural protein 2 inhibits type I/II interferon-stimulated JAK-STAT signaling. J Virol 84: 10877–10887.

Chapter 6

Co-infection with Dengue and Chikungunya Viruses

Farah Deeba, Nazia Afreen, Asimul Islam, Irshad Hussain Naqvi, Shobha Broor, Anwar Ahmed and Shama Parveen

Additional information is available at the end of the chapter

http://dx.doi.org/10.5772/64308

Abstract

Dengue and Chikungunya fever are the arboviral infections that are endemic in tropical and subtropical regions. These two viral infections share common clinical symptoms. These infections are transmitted by a common mosquito vector so these viruses co-circulate in many geographical regions. Various clinical investigations, particularly from India and African countries have documented the dual infection with these viruses. However, the true disease burden of Dengue and Chikungunya dual viral infections is still not known because most of these studies involved a smaller patient group. Therefore, in depth investigations involving larger patient groups are needed to examine the complete pathogenicity and severity of the dual viral infections. The timely diagnosis of the pathogens and correlation of disease severity with mono or dual infections is essential for effective patient management. In addition, the detailed molecular and cellular mechanism of co-infection should be investigated to describe a complete picture of the interaction of two viral pathogens in the host cell. Further comprehensive studies of dual infections from the endemic regions will determine the epidemiological and evolutionary pattern of these emerging viruses. This data will also assist in designing and implementation of effective control measures.

Keywords: Chikungunya virus, Dengue virus, co-infections, *Aedes* mosquito

1. Introduction

Both Dengue and Chikungunya fever are arboviral infections of global importance. The two diseases share a common mode of transmission, i.e. through different species of mosquitoes. Therefore, these infections are normally present in the same geographical locations. Dengue virus belongs to family Flaviviridae and genus Flavivirus. It is a small enveloped RNA virus carrying a single stranded, positive-sense RNA genome of 10.6 kb in length. Dengue virus exists as four serotypes (DENV 1-4) which offer only transient cross protection to each other

[1]. Four to five genotypes are distinguished within each serotype of the dengue virus. The Chikungunya virus (CHIKV) belongs to the Togaviridae family and genus Alphavirus. It has a linear positive sense RNA genome of 1.8 Kb in length. Three genotypes (Eastern, Central South African [ECSA], West African and Asian) have been described for the Chikungunya virus [2,3]. Laboratory diagnosis of the two viral infections is done by virus isolation, genome detection (RT-PCR) and antibody detection (IgM or IgG ELISA). In addition, the antigen detection (NS1 ELISA) is also being used for diagnosis of Dengue viral infection. No licensed vaccine is available against these arboviral diseases. In addition, no antiviral drug has been developed against these viruses.

Due to many common clinical presentations, Chikungunya fever is often misdiagnosed with Dengue viral infection. As Dengue fever has a high incidence rate, the symptomatic patients are tested for Dengue virus only and rarely for Chikungunya viral infection. Thus the patients suspected with Dengue and/or Chikungunya virus infection should be tested for both the viruses especially in the endemic areas. This is essential for accurate and timely diagnosis of the viral infection that will assist in appropriate patient management. Therefore, regular surveillance for both the viruses should be done in the endemic areas. This will assist in the prediction and control of the outbreaks. The molecular characterization of the circulating strains of the Dengue and Chikungunya viruses is done by DNA sequencing followed by phylogenetic analysis. Description of the circulating strains is essential to study the epidemiology of these rapidly evolving viruses [4,5,6]. In addition, this information is essential for designing the strategies to control the epidemics.

2. Clinical manifestations

Both Dengue and Chikungunya viral infections have many common clinical presentations like high grade fever, headache, nausea, rashes and body pain. In case of a mild infection, the viral titre decreases in around 10 days and the symptoms subside because these are the self limiting infections. But when there is a severe dengue infection, it causes bleeding in DHF (dengue hemorrhagic fever) and/or shock caused by plasma leakage in DSS (dengue shock syndrome). The most prominent feature of Chikungunya infection is the severe joint pain which sometimes can persist for a few months to a year. A severe Chikungunya viral infection can cause neurological and optical manifestations. Thus, Chikungunya viral infection is usually non-fatal while Dengue fever may result in severe complications including death. Therefore, co-infection with the two viruses may result in disease with overlapping symptoms. Hence, the diagnosis and treatment of such patients become difficult. Therefore, this issue of clinical manifestations in case of dual infections with the two viruses should be addressed adequately. Hence, the timely diagnosis of the dual infections is essential for better patient management.

Limited investigations have studied the role of dual viral infections in clinical presentation of the disease. According to a recent investigation, patients having co-infection with the Dengue and Chikungunya viruses present a clinically severe disease with a high mortality rate when compared to mono-infection with these viruses [7]. The requirement of mechanical ventilation and blood transfusion was found to be higher in the co-infected patients. Chahar and colleagues also reported the involvement of central nervous system and hemorrhagic manifestations in two out of six co-infected patients and one death [8]. In contrast, another study from Africa compared the clinical symptoms of 19 Chikungunya and Dengue virus co-infected patients and it was concluded that the co-infection was also not associated with any particular clinical manifestations [9]. Further elaborate investigations involving larger patient group are needed to understand the complete pathogenesis and severity of the dual viral infections.

3. The vector

The main vector for the transmission of Dengue and Chikungunya viral infection is *Aedes aegypti.* Another species of mosquito, the *Aedes albopictus* act as the secondary vector for the transmission of both the viral infections. The *Aedes albopictus* emerged as highly competent vector for the transmission of Chikungunya viral infection during the massive outbreak in 2004 in the Indian Ocean [10]. The *Aedes albopictus* appeared to be an efficient vector for replication of a mutated strain of Chikungunya virus with a change in Alanine to Valine at 226 position of the E1 glycoprotein (E1-A226V) during this epidemic [11]. The *Aedes albopictus* commonly known as the Asian tiger mosquito is a tropical and subtropical vector. The overall geographical distribution of *Aedes* mosquitoes has changed since this outbreak. The *Aedes albopictus* is now spreading to regions that were earlier inhabited by the *Aedes aegypti.* Consequently, the circulation patterns of the Dengue and Chikungunya viruses as well as the dynamics of the epidemics caused by these viruses are expected to be modified in future [12].

4. Dengue and Chikungunya virus co-infection in the vector

It has been postulated that two different viruses cause dual infection of a mosquito vector by consecutive bites of two different infected human patients or by a single bite of a co-infected patient. Furthermore, a concurrent viral infection in humans occur due to bite of a mosquito that is infected with both the viruses or bites with two different mosquitoes each infected with a separate virus. Limited investigations are available on the role of vectors in disease transmission because of lack of technical expertise and limited resources of vector surveillance in the endemic areas. *Aedes albopictus* has been shown to have the ability of getting orally co-infected with Dengue and Chikungunya virus [13]. The study reported that both Dengue and Chikungunya viruses were able to replicate simultaneously in the mosquito and have the ability to deliver concomitantly infectious particles of Dengue and Chikungunya virus in a single bite via saliva. In addition, a secondary infection with the Chikungunya virus could be introduced in mosquitoes that had a primary infection with Dengue virus. Another recent study showed simultaneous infection, dissemination and transmission of Dengue and Chikungunya virus in the two mosquito species, *Aedes aegypti* and *Aedes albopictus* [14]. In this study, groups of mosquitoes were orally infected with Dengue and Chikungunya virus simultaneously or sequentially. Mosquitoes were then tested for their potential to disseminate and transmit both the viruses simultaneously by quantitative RT-PCR. Simultaneous dissemination of Dengue and Chikungunya virus was detected in both the species of the mosquitoes. The authors observed a lower rate of dissemination of both the viruses when administered simultaneously as compared to the sequential infection in which a significantly higher rate of dissemination of both the viruses was found.

Earlier studies have suggested that vector competence of the mosquito may depend on the type and the genetic makeup of infecting viral strain. An investigation from France stated that *Aedes albopictus* was more competent for Chikungunya virus as compared to the Dengue-2 virus. The virus replicated to high levels in the mosquito species and could be transmitted from mosquito as early as 2 days after ingestion of infected blood by the mosquito with 1000 viral RNA molecules in the salivary glands [15]. Similarly, another study from Thailand also concluded that the rate of multiplication and oral receptivity of the Chikungunya virus was faster in laboratory-bred *Aedes aegepti* as compared to the Dengue virus [16]. *Aedes albopictus* was proved to be an efficient vector for dissemination and transmission of the Chikungunya virus as compared to *Aedes aegypti* [10]. A single amino acid mutation in the Chikungunya virus genome (E1-A226V) resulted in increased fitness of the virus in *Aedes albopictus*. This probably caused enhanced transmission of the Chikungunya virus by *Aedes albopictus* which further resulted in the massive outbreak in the Indian Ocean. The complete mechanism of co-infection of mosquitoes with two different arboviruses should be investigated further using different viral strains. The elucidation of detailed molecular and cellular events involved in such co-infections will have an impact on prediction and control of the viral outbreaks.

5. Dengue and Chikungunya virus co-infection: *in vitro* studies

Co-infection of the two viruses has been studied *in vitro* also using *Aedes albopictus* C6/36 cell line [17]. In this study the DENV-3 and Chikungunya virus (ECSA genotype) isolated from the infected mosquitoes was used to characterize their co-infection. The duplex -RT-PCR (D-RT-PCR) technique was used to determine virus production. The D-RT-PCR was positive for both the viruses when an equal multiplicity of infection (MOI) or a higher MOI for Chikungunya virus was used. But when a higher titer of DENV- 3 was used, the D-RT-PCR was positive only for DENV-3. Thus, the authors concluded that higher titer of Dengue-3 virus resulted in competitive suppression of the replication of Chikungunya virus. They also reported that both viruses' replications depend on virus titer and not on serial infection. Further elaborate investigations are needed to describe a complete picture of the interaction of the two viral pathogens in the host cell.

6. Dengue and Chikungunya virus co-infection in humans

Due to common vectors, Dengue and Chikungunya viruses can co-infect a human host. This has been documented in several studies from India and Africa (Table 1) (Figure 1 and 2). The first documented case of Dengue and Chikungunya virus co-infection in humans was reported as early as 1967. The two viruses were isolated from a patient seen in Vellore, South India [18]. The patient also showed an increase in antibodies against Dengue and Chikungunya virus in serial blood samples. Subsequently co-infection of Dengue and Chikungunya has been

http://dx.doi.org/10.5772/64308

reported in many studies from India, but the proportion of co-infected cases vary in different studies ranging from 0.1 to 23% (Figure 2).

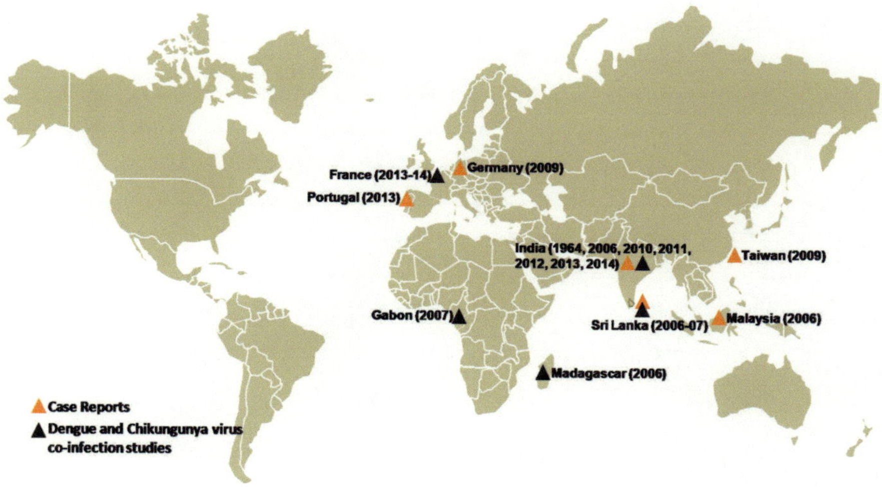

Figure 1. The world map showing co-infection with Dengue and Chikungunya viruses in different geographical regions. The freely available world map was downloaded from the website, presentationmagazine.com (http://www.presentationmagazine.com/world-maps-vectoreditable-507.htm). The map was created and edited in PowerPoint.

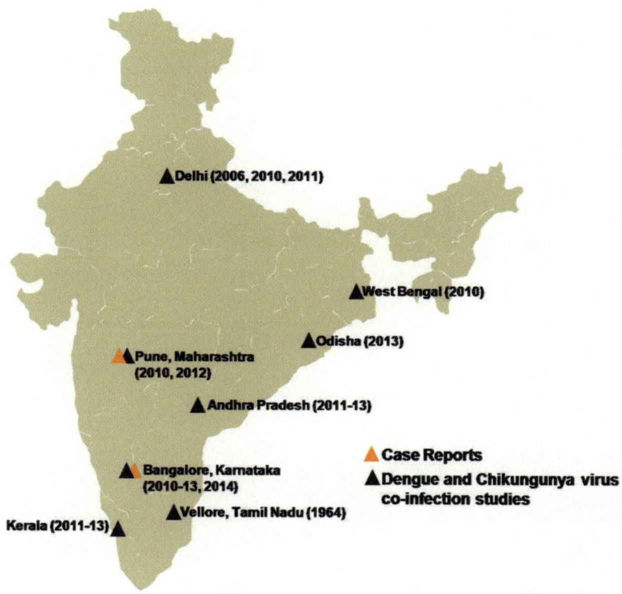

Figure 2. The map of India showing co-infection with Dengue and Chikungunya viruses. The map was downloaded from the website, presentationmagazine.com (http://www.presentationmagazine.com/world-maps-vector-editable-507.htm). The map was created and edited in PowerPoint.

Study site (Year)	No of samples tested	Method (DFA/culture/ ELISA/PCR)	**No of Virus +ve (%)**	**Dengue virus +ve (%)**	**Chikungunya virus +ve (%)**	**Co-infections**	**Reference**
Vellore, India (1964)	372	ELISA	206 (55)	11(3)	202 (54)	7 (2)	[14]
Delhi, India (2006)	69	RT-PCR	65 (94)	48 (70)	17 (25)	6 (9)	[4]
Delhi, India (2010)	432	RT-PCR	93 (22)	54 (13)	39 (9)	5 (1)	[15]
Delhi, India (2011)	87	RT-PCR	59 (68)	43 (49)	25 (29)	9 (10)	[16]
Odisha, India (2013)	204	ELISA	124 (56)	96 (47)	72 (32)	43 (19)	[17]
Kerala, Andhra Pradesh, India (2011-13)	1024	ELISA and RT-PCR	249 (24.3)	194 (18.9)	55 (5)	25 (2.4)	[18]
Bangalore, India (2010-13)	6554	ELISA	3824 (58)	3202 (49)	622 (10)	532 (8)	[19]
Pune, India (2010)	364	ELISA	175 (48)	121 (33)	79 (22)	25 (7)	[3]
West Bengal, India (2010)	550	ELISA	303 (55)	172 (31)	199 (36)	68 (12)	[21]
Gabon, Africa (2007)	773	RT-PCR	329 (43)	54 (7)	275 (36)	8 (1)	[8]
Gabon, Africa (2007)	4287	RT-PCR		367 (9)	1567 (37)	37 (0.9)	[5]
Madagascar, Africa (2006)	55	RT-PCR	38 (69)	24(44%)	4(7%)	10 (0.2)	[24]
Saint Martin, France (2013-14)	1502	RT-PCR and ELISA	635 (42)	65 (4)	570 (38)	16 (2.8)	[22]
Sri Lanka	54		41(76)	20 (37)	21(39)	3 (5.5)	[23]

Table 1. Studies on co-infections with Dengue and Chikungunya viruses

Chahar and colleagues conducted Dengue and Chikungunya virus specific RT-PCR on patients suspected of Dengue and/or Chikungunya fever in New Delhi, India [8]. Their study detected 6 (8.7%) co-infected patients. All 6 patients had fever, headache, joint pain, and low thrombocyte counts (<100,000/mm^3). Two of the co-infected patients had dengue hemorrhagic fever with central nervous system (CNS) involvement. In another study from Delhi, 5 (1.1%) co-infection cases were detected in the samples tested by RT-PCR [19]. All the co-infecting strains clustered with genotype II of Dengue 1 virus and ECSA genotype of the Chikungunya virus on phylogenetic analysis. Concurrent infection with the Dengue and Chikungunya viruses were detected in 9 (10%) samples tested by RT-PCR in a recent study from our laboratory from New Delhi, India [20]. Genetic characterization of the co-infecting strains showed that CHIKV belonged to East Central South African genotype and Dengue strains belonged to the American African genotype of DENV-1. Co-infection with the two viruses was detected in 28 (13.7%) of the samples by RT-PCR in a recent study from Odisha, India [21]. Dayakar and co-workers [22] have recently reported co-infection by Dengue and Chikungunya viruses in 23% of the suspected patients by RT-PCR from Andhra Pradesh and 0.1 % from Kerala in Southern part of India. Sheikh and colleagues carried out IgM ELISA specific for Dengue and Chikungunya virus on samples collected from Karnataka, India [23]. Specific antibodies against both Dengue and Chikungunya virus were detected in 532 (8.1%) samples. Another investigation from Tirupati, a Southern part of India detected anibodies in 2 (2.7%) of the samples tested by IgM ELISA [24]. Gandhi and co-workers [7] have identified dual infection with Chikungunya and Dengue viruses in 25 (6.8%) of the patients by IgM ELISA from Pune. Dual infections with both the viruses were reported in 68 (12.4%) samples by IgM ELISA from West Bengal, an Eastern part of India [25].

Various investigations from different geographical regions have also described the co-infections with the two viruses (Figure 1), including 2.8% in France [26], 5.5% in Sri Lanka [27]. A serological study from Sri Lanka reported co-infection with the two viruses in 3 (5.5%) of the samples tested by IgM ELISA [27]. Various African countries have reported co-infection with the two viruses. Chikungunya and Dengue viruses caused a large simultaneous outbreak in southeast Gabon in Central Africa in 2010. Between 2007 and 2010, a total of 4287 acutely febrile patients were investigated for both the viral infections by quantitative real-time reverse-transcription polymerase reaction [9]. Out of the samples tested, 1567 were CHIKV-positive, 376 DENV-2–positive, and 37 (0.9%) co-infected. When a human case of co-infection was diagnosed in the above mentioned study, mosquitoes were captured around the patient's home during daytime. One CHIKV- and DENV-2–coinfected *A.albopictus* specimen was also detected in the study, which represented the first observation of dual mosquito infection in nature. Detection of co-infection of Dengue and Chikungunya virus in *A.albopictus* demonstrates the possibility that humans could be co-infected with the 2 viruses by the bite of a single mosquito. Viral loads were determined for the 24 co-infected, 121 CHIKV-positive and 52 DENV-2– positive patients. Mean values of Dengue and Chikungunya viral loads in co-infected patients were significantly lower than mean values in CHIKV- and DENV-2–mono infected patients. Thus, the investigators concluded that the two viruses exerted a suppression effect on each other. Phylogenetic analysis revealed that the CHIKV and DENV-2 isolates belonged to African clusters and they grouped together with strains reported from other parts of Africa. In another study from the same region, the samples were tested by real time RT-PCR and 8 (1%) were co-infections [12]. In another investigation conducted in Madagascar, another African country, dengue like cases were investigated by RT-PCR and ELISA. Ten (18%) samples were found to be co-infected by both Dengue and Chikungunya virus [28].

Simultaneous detection of the two viruses has been described in a number of case reports (Table 2) (Figure 1 and 2). A case report identified Dengue and Chikungunya viruses in an eight year old child at Mysore in Southern part of India [29]. Raut and colleagues recently reported a case of multiple co-infections in a young man after his return from Nigeria [30]. The patient was positive for dengue xlink antigen as well as Dengue and Chikungunya virus by RT-PCR. Apart from Dengue and Chikungunya virus, the patient was also positive for the malarial parasite, *Plasmodium falciparum*. A recent investigation reported that a woman returning to Portugal from Angola was infected with Dengue 4 virus and ECSA genotype of the Chikungunya virus [31]. Another case of imported infection in patients who had returned to Taiwan from Singapore was reported [32]. Dengue and Chikungunya virus co-infection in this patient was confirmed by real time PCR and sero conversion for both the viruses in the convalescent-phase serum samples. The co-infecting viruses were identified as the Dengue virus serotype 2 and ECSA genotype of the Chikungunya virus. Dual infection with both the viruses was detected in a German traveler who was employed as a social worker in India [33]. Two different patients had infection with the two viruses in Malaysia [34]. An 80 year old patient from Sri Lanka was diagnosed with Dengue and Chikungunya virus infection by RT-PCR [35].

Study site (Year)	Age of patient (in Years)	Co-Infecting pathogens	Reference
Malaysia (2006)	Case 1: 28 Case 2: 22	DENV+CHIKV	[30]
Sri Lanka (2006)	70	DENV+CHIKV	[31]
Germany (2009)	25	DENV+CHIKV	[29]
Taiwan (2009)	12	DENV-2 +CHIKV	[28]
India (2012)	8	DENV+CHIKV	[25]
Portugal (2013)	50+	DENV-4+CHIKV	[27]
India (2014)	21	DENV+CHIKV+ *Plasmodium falciparum*	[26]

Table 2. Case studies involving Co-infections with Dengue and Chikungunya viruses

Additionally, the latest information of the ongoing outbreaks of these two arboviruses is available on the WHO/CDC/PAHO websites. The interactive map of recent and ongoing Chikungunya fever outbreaks is available at: http://www.arcgis.com/apps/MapTools/index.html?appid=ce2372254ce743b79d332b43724cd9e5 and Dengue map, a CDC- health map collaboration is available at: http://www.healthmap.org/dengue/en/. These interactive maps report recent Dengue and Chikungunya outbreaks throughout the world and global risk areas. The map shows recent reports of local and imported cases based on official, newspapers and other media sources. Global risk areas are determined by consensus between sources including: national surveillance systems, published literature, questionnaires and formal and informal news reports.

Detection of high number of co-infection cases in some of the studies mentioned above shows that many Chikungunya cases go undiagnosed in Dengue endemic regions, thereby concealing the true burden of the Chikungunya viral infection. Further epidemiological and viral investigations involving larger patient group in the endemic areas are needed to define the precise role of Dengue and Chikungunya viruses in clinical presentation of these dual

http://dx.doi.org/10.5772/64308

infections. These studies will further assist to monitor the spread of these arboviruses and implementation of appropriate control strategies.

7. Dengue, Chikungunya and Zika virus co-infection in humans

Zika virus (ZIKV) is also an arbovirus and a member of Flaviviridae family. It was first identified in rhesus monkey in Zika forests of Uganda in 1947 [36]. The mode of transmission of Zika virus is same as for Dengue and Chikungunya viruses, i.e., through *Aedes spp*. The non-mosquito mediated transmission of ZIKV include sexual and mother to fetus transmission during pregnancy [37, 38]. The febrile illness due to Zika virus is very much overlapping with that of Chikungunya and Dengue virus Infections [39]. High grade fever, arthralgia, myalgia, retro-orbital pain etc are a few common symptoms. Subsequently, after a few sporadic cases of ZIKV in Africa, the first documented epidemic in Yap Island occurred in 2007 affecting more than half of the population in Yap Island [40]. Similarly outbreaks of ZIKV were reported from Pacific islands including French Polynesia, New Caledonia, Cook Islands, Easter islands, etc in 2013-14 that affected thousands of inhabitants [41]. In 2015 the largest epidemic of Zika virus started in Brazil that later spread to other American countries and Caribbean region affecting millions of people [42]. The Zika virus infection during ongoing pandemic is also found to be associated with many neurological complications like Guillain-Barré syndrome and microcephaly [43]. A recent report suggested that till 6 April 2016, 62 countries [44] (mostly in South and North America) have reported active transmission of ZIKV. Additionally, the virus has also been detected in returning travelers from 13 non-endemic countries [45-49].

Thus currently, the Zika virus is co-circulating with Chikungunya virus in many parts of world including Americas [36]. Recently in 2015 Villamil-Gomez and coworkers reported co-infection with Dengue, Chikungunya and Zika viruses in a 49 year old male patient from Columbia. The patient was reported with febrile illness with 38^0C temperature, conjuctivitis, maculopopular rashes etc,. The blood sample collected from the patient was positive for Dengue and Chikungunya virus IgM antibodies. Additionally, the sample was positive by RT-PCR for ZIKV and DENV [50, 51]. The authors observed no synergistic effect of these infections in the patient [50]. Therefore, differential diagnosis of these arboviral infections should be done on patients during the ongoing ZIKV pandemic in this region for proper patient management. Subsequent detailed investigations will determine the affect of co-infections with these arboviruses on disease severity.

8. Conclusions

Dengue and Chikungunya viruses can cause dual infections in humans and in the mosquito vector. The significance of the Dengue and Chikungunya dual viral infections can be elucidated by measuring viral loads of each infecting virus and the effect of competitive suppression of the infecting viruses. Further investigations are needed on transmissibility studies in the mosquitoes using chimeric viruses. In addition, more elaborate clinical studies involving larger patient groups are required to ascertain the effect of severity of the disease in case of dual viral infections. Also, the clinically suspected cases should be tested for both the pathogens in the endemic areas. This information is essential for early and timely diagnosis of the infecting pathogen and correlation of the clinical symptoms with mono or dual infections for appropriate patient management. It has been postulated that a recent increase in Dengue and Chikungunya virus co-infection may affect the evolution of these rapidly emerging viruses. In addition, the infectivity as well as the pathogenicity of these viruses may also be affected in future. Further, continuous surveillance for both Dengue and Chikungunya viruses is essential in the endemic areas for identification and characterization of these viral pathogens. This information will also help in the implementation of proper measures to control the outbreaks caused by these emerging viral pathogens.

Acknowledgements

We acknowledge the financial support of University Grants Commission and Council of Scientific and Industrial Research, Government of India.

Author details

Farah Deeba[1 #], Nazia Afreen[1 #], Asimul Islam[1], Irshad Hussain Naqvi[2], Shobha Broor[3], Anwar Ahmed[4] and Shama Parveen[1*]

*Address all correspondence to: shamp25@yahoo.com, sparveen2@jmi.ac.in

1 Centre for Interdisciplinary Research in Basic Sciences, Jamia Millia Islamia, New Delhi, India

2 Dr. M.A. Ansari Health Centre, Jamia Millia Islamia, New Delhi, India

3 Department of Microbiology, Faculty of Medicine and Health Science, Shree Guru Gobind Singh Tricentenary University, Haryana, India

4 Protein Research Chair, Department of Biochemistry, College of Science, King Saud University, Riyadh, Saudi Arabia

[#]These Authors contrubuted equally to this work.

References

[1] Heinz FX & Stiasny K. Flaviviruses and flavivirus vaccines. Vaccine. 2012; 30(29): 4301–4306.

[2] Santhosh SR, Dash PK, Parida MM, Khan M, Tiwari M, Rao PVL. Comparative full genome analysis revealed E1: A226V shift in 2007 Indian Chikungunya virus isolates. Vir Res. 2008; 135:36–41.

[3] Deeba F, Islam A, Kazim SN, Naqvi IH, Broor S, Ahmed A and Parveen S. Chikungunya virus: recent advances in epidemiology, host pathogen interaction and vaccine strategies. Pathogens and Disease. 2016, 74(3).

[4] Afreen N, Deeba F, Naqvi IH, Shareef M, Ahmed A, Broor S, and Parveen S. Molecular Investigation of 2013 Dengue Fever Outbreak from Delhi, India. Version 1. PLoS Curr. 2014, 2(6): ecurrents.outbreaks. 0411252a8b82aa933f6540abb54a855f.

[5] Afreen N, Naqvi IH, Broor S, Ahmed A, Parveen S. Phylogenetic and Molecular Clock Analysis of Dengue Serotype 1 and 3 from New Delhi, India. PLoS ONE. 2015;10(11): e0141628.

[6] Afreen N, Naqvi IH, Broor S, Ahmed A, Kazim SN, Dohare R, Kumar M, Parveen S. Evolutionary 1 analysis of Dengue serotype 2 viruses using Phylogenetic and Bayesian methods from New Delhi, India. PloS Negl Trop Dis. 2016; 10(3): e0004511.

[7] Gandhi BS, Kulkarni K, Godbole M, Dole SS, Kapur S, Satpathy P, Khatri AM, Deshpande PS, Azad F, Gupte N, Bharadwaj R, Bollinger RC and Gupta A. Dengue and Chikungunya co-infection associated with more severe clinical disease than mono-infection. International J. of Healthcare and Biomedical Research. 2015; 3(3):117-123.

[8] Chahar HS, Bharaj P, Dar L, Guleria R, Kabra SK and Broor S. Co-infections with chikungunya virus and dengue virus in Delhi, India. Emerging infectious diseases. 2009; 15(7):1077–80.

[9] Caron M, Paupy C, Grard G, Becquart P, Mombo I, Nso BB, Kassa Kassa F, Nkoghe D, Leroy EM. Recent introduction and rapid dissemination of Chikungunya virus and dengue virus serotype 2 associated with human and mosquito coinfections in Gabon, Central Africa. Clinical Infectious Diseases. 2012; 55(6):45–53.

[10] Tsetsarkin KA, Vanlandingham DL, McGee CE, Higgs S. A single mutation in Chikungunya virus affects vector specificity and epidemic potential. PLOS Pathog. 2007; 3(12):e201.

[11] Schuffenecker I, Iteman I, Michault A, Murri S, Frangeul L, Vaney MC, Lavenir R, Pardigon N, Reynes JM, Pettinelli, Biscornet L, Diancourt L, Michel S, Duquerroy S, Guigon G, Frenkiel MP, Brehin AC, Cubito N, Despre P, Kunst F, Rey FA, Zeller H and Brisse S. Genome microevolution of Chikungunya viruses causing the Indian Ocean outbreak. PLoS Med. 2006; 3(7): e263.

[12] Leroy EM, Nkoghe D, Ollomo B, Nze-Nkogue C, Becquart P, Grard G, Pourrut X, Charrel R, Moureau G, Ndjoyi-Mbiguino A and Lamballerie XD. Concurrent Chikungunya and Dengue virus infections during simultaneous outbreaks, Gabon, 2007. Emerg. Infect. Dis. 2009; 15(40): 591-593.

[13] Vazeille M, Mousson L, Martin E, Failloux A-B. Orally Co-Infected Aedes albopictus from La Reunion Island, Indian Ocean, Can Deliver Both Dengue and Chikungunya Infectious Viral Particles in Their Saliva. PLoS Negl Trop Dis. 2010; 4(6): e706.

[14] Nuckols JT, Huang Y-JS, Higgs S, Miller AL, Pyles RB, Spratt HM, Horne KM and Vanlandingham DL. Evaluation of Simultaneous Transmission of Chikungunya Virus and Dengue Virus Type 2 in Infected Aedes aegypti and Aedes albopictus (Diptera: Culicidae). Journal of Medical Entomology. 2015; 52(3), pp.447–451.

[15] Moutailler S, Barre H, Vazeille M and Failloux AB. Recently introduced Aedes albopictus in Corsica is competent to Chikungunya virus and in a lesser extent to dengue virus. Trop. Med. Intl.Health. 2009; 14: 1105–1109.

[16] Rohani A, Potiwat R, Zamree I, and Lee HL. Refractoriness of Aedes aegypti (Linnaeus) to dual infection with dengue and chikungunya virus. Southeast Asian J. Trop. Med. Public Health. 2009; 40: 443–448.

[17] Potiwat R, Komalamisra N, Thavara U, Tawatsin A, Siriyasatien P. Competitive Suppression between Chikungunya and Dengue virus in Aedes albopictus C6 / 36. SouthEast Asian Journal of Tropical Medicine and Public Health. 2011; 42(6):1388–1394.

[18] Myers RM & Carey DE. Concurrent isolation from patient of two arboviruses, chikungunya and dengue type 2. Science. 1967; *157*(3794), 1307-1308.

[19] Singh P, Mittal V, Rizvi MM, Chhabra M, Sharma P, Rawat DS, Bhattacharya D, Chauhan LS, Rai A. The first dominant co-circulation of both dengue and Chikungunya viruses during the post-monsoon period of 2010 in Delhi, India. Epidem Infect. 2012; 140:1337–1342.

[20] Afreen N, Deeba F, Khan WH, Haider SH, Kazim SN, Ishrat R, Naqvi IH, Shareef MY, Broor S, Ahmed A and Parveen S. Molecular characterization of dengue and chikungunya virus strains circulating in New Delhi, India. Microbiology and Immunology. 2014; 58:688–696.

[21] Saswat T, Kumar A, Kumar S, Mamidi P, Muduli S, Debata NK, Pal NS, Pratheek BM, Chattopadhyay S, and Chattopadhyay S. High rates of co-infection of Dengue and Chikungunya virus in Odisha and Maharashtra, India during 2013. Infection, Genetics and Evolution. 2015. doi: http://dx.doi.org/10.1016/j.meegid.2015.08.006

[22] Dayakar S, Goud IK, Pillai H, Remadevi V, Dharmaseelan S, Nair RR, Pillai MR. Molecular Diagnosis of Chikungunya virus (CHIKV) and Dengue virus (DENV) and its concomitant circulation in South Indian population. Virology Reports. 2015; pp.1–7. http://dx.doi.org/10.1016/j.virep.2015.05.001.

[23] Shaikh N, Raut CG, Manjunatha M. Co-infections with chikungunya and dengue viruses®: A serological study in Karnataka state, India. Indian journal of Medical Microbiology. 2015; 33(3):459–460.

[24] Kalawat U, Sharma KK, Reddy SG. Prevalence of dengue and Chikungunya fever and their co-infection. Indian J Pathol Mirobiol. 2011; 54: 844-6.

[25] Taraphdar D, Sarkar A, Mukhopadhyay BB, Chatterjee S. A comparative study of clinical features between monotypic and dual infection cases with Chikungunya virus and dengue virus in West Bengal, India. Am J Trop Med Hyg. 2012; 86:720–723.

[26] Omarjee R, Prat C, Flusin O, Boucau S, Tenebray B, Merle O, Huc-Anais P, Cassadou S, Leparc-Goffart I. Importance of case definition to monitor ongoing outbreak of chikungunya virus on a background of actively circulating dengue virus, St Martin, December 2013 to January 2014. Eurosurveillance. 2014; 19(13).

[27] Kularatne SAM, Gihan MC, Weerasinghe SC, Gunasena S. Concurrent outbreaks of Chikungunya and Dengue fever in Kandy, Sri Lanka, 2006–07: a comparative analysis of clinical and laboratory features. Postgrad Med J. 2009; 85:342–346.

[28] Ratsitorahina M, Harisoa J, Ratovonjato J, Biacabe S, Reynes J-M, Zeller H, Raoelina Y, Talarmin A, Richard V and Soares JL. Outbreak of Dengue and Chikungunya fevers,Toamasina, Madagascar, 2006. Emerg Infect Dis. 2008; 14 (7):1135-1137.

[29] Kumar KJ, Manjunath VG, Shailashree M, Girish GN. Coinfection with dengue and Chikungunya--a case report. J Indian Med Assoc. 2012; 110(10):749,752.

[30] Raut CG, Rao NM, Sinha DP, Hanumaiah H, Manjunatha MJ. Malaria Co-Infection after Travel to Nigeria, India Chikungunya Virus Outbreak, Dominica, 2014. Emerging infectious diseases. 2015; 21(5):908–909.

[31] Parreira R, Centeno-Lima S, Lopes A, Portugal-Calisto D, Constantino A, Nina J. Dengue virus serotype 4 and Chikungunya virus coinfection in a traveler returning from Luanda, Angola, January 2014. Eurosurveillance. 2014; 19(10):6–9.

[32] Chang SF, Su CL, Shu PY, Yang CF, Liao TL, Cheng CH, Hu HC and Huang JH. Concurrent Isolation of Chikungunya Virus and Dengue Virus from a Patient with Coinfection Resulting from a Trip to Singapore. J of Clinical Microbiology. 2010; 48(12): 4586–4589.

[33] Schilling S, Emmerich P, Gunther S and Schmidt-Chanasit J. Dengue and Chikungunya virus co-infection in a German traveler. J of Clin Virol. 2009; *45:163–164.*

[34] Nayar SK, Noridah O, Paranthaman V, Ranjit K, Norizah I, Chem YK, Mustafa B, Chua KB. Co-infection of dengue virus and Chikungunya virus in two patients with acute febrile illness. Med J Malaysia, 2007; 62(4):335-6.

[35] Hapuarachchi HAC, Bandara KBAT, Hapugoda MD, Williams S and Abeyewickreme W. Laboratory confirmation of dengue and chikungunya co-infection. Ceylon Medical Journal. 2008; 53 (3): 104-5.

[36] Dick G. Zika virus (II). Pathogenicity and physical properties. Transactions of the Royal Society of Tropical Medicine and Hygiene. 1952; 46:521-534.

[37] Mansuy JM, Dutertre M, Mengelle C, Fourcade C, Marchou B, Delobel P, Izopet J, and Martin-Blondel G. "Zika virus: high infectious viral load in semen, a new sexually transmitted pathogen." Lancet Infect Dis. 2016;16(405): 00138-00139.

[38] Petersen LR, Jamieson DJ, Powers AM & Honein MA. Zika Virus. New England Journal of Medicine. 2016. DOI: 10.1056/NEJMra1602113

[39] Pastula DM, Smith DE, Beckham DJ & Tyler KL. Four emerging arboviral diseases in North America: Jamestown Canyon, Powassan, chikungunya, and Zika virus diseases. J. Neurovirol. 2016. DOI 10.1007/s13365-016-0428-5.

[40] Duffy MR, Chen TH, Hancock WT, Powers AM, Kool JL, Lanciotti RS, Pretrick M, Marfel M, Holzbauer S, Dubray C, Guillaumot L, Griggs A, Bel M, Lambert AJ,Laven J, Kosoy O, Panella A, Biggerstaff BJ, Fischer M, Hayes EB. Zika virus outbreak on Yap Island, federated states of Micronesia. New England Journal of Medicine. 2009; 360: 2536-2543.

[41] Cauchemez S, Besnard M, Bompard P, Dub T, Guillemette-Artur P, Eyrolle-Guignot D, Salje H, Van Kerkhove MD, Abadie V, Garel C, Fontanet A, Mallet HP. Association between Zika virus and microcephaly in French Polynesia, 2013–15: a retrospective study. The Lancet (2016). doi: 10.1016/S0140-6736(16)00651-6.

[42] Cardoso CW, Paploski IAD, Kikuti M, Rodrigues MS, Silva MMO, Campos GS, Sardi SI, Kitron U, Reis MG, Ribeiro GS. Outbreak of Exanthematous Illness Associated with Zika, Chikungunya, and Dengue Viruses, Salvador, Brazil. Emerging Infectious Diseases. 2015; 21(12): 2274-6.

[43] CDC "Zika Virus" Website. Available via: http://www.cdc.gov/zika/. [Accessed: 2016-04-10]

[44] Organisation, W. H. (2016). "ZIKA VIRUS, Microcephaly and Guillain-Barré Syndrome :Situation Report, 7 April 2016." from http://apps.who.int/iris/bitstream/10665/204961/1/zikasitrep_7Apr2016_eng.pdf?ua=1

[45] Zammarchi, L, Tappe D, Fortuna C, Remoli M, Gunther S, Venturi G, Bartoloni A, Schmidt-Chanasit J. Zika virus infection in a traveller returning to Europe from Brazil, March 2015. EuroSurveill. 2015; 20: 10.2807.

[46] Kutsuna S, Kato Y, Takasaki T, Moi M, Kotaki A, Uemura H, Matono T, Fujiya Y, Mawatari M, Takeshita N. Two cases of Zika fever imported from French Polynesia to Japan, December 2013 to January 2014. Euro Surveill. 2014;19:1-5.

[47] Kwong JC, Druce JD & Leder K. Zika virus infection acquired during brief travel to Indonesia. The American journal of tropical medicine and hygiene. 2013;89: 516-517.

[48] Fonseca K, Meatherall B, Zarra D, Drebot M, MacDonald J, Pabbaraju K, Wong S, Webster P, Lindsay R, Tellier R. First case of Zika virus infection in a returning Canadian traveler. The American journal of tropical medicine and hygiene. 2014;91:1035-1038.

[49] Foy BD, Kobylinski KC, Chilson Foy JL, Blitvich BJ, Travassos da Rosa A, Haddow AD, Lanciotti RS, Tesh RB. Probable non-vector-borne transmission of Zika virus, Colorado, USA. Emerg Infect Dis. 2011;17:880-2.

[50] Villamil-Gomez WE, Gonzalez-Camargo O, Rodriguez-Ayubi J, Zapata-Serpa D, Rodriguez-Morales AJ. Dengue, chikungunya and Zika co-infection in a patient from Colombia. J Infect Public Health (2015). http://dx.doi.org/10.1016/j.jiph.2015.12.002.

[51] Villamil-Gómez WE, Rodriguez-Morales AJ. Reply: Dengue RT-PCR-positive, Chikungunya IgM-positive and Zika RT-PCR-positive co-infection in a patient from Colombia. J Infect Public Health (2016). http://dx.doi.org/10.1016/j.jiph.2016.02.003.

Section 2

Entomology

Chapter 7

Vector Control in Chikungunya and Other Arboviruses

Sengodan Karthi and Muthugounder Subramaniam Shivakumar

Additional information is available at the end of the chapter

http://dx.doi.org/10.5772/63134

Abstract

Mosquito vectors are solely responsible for transmitting diseases, such as malaria, yellow fever, chikungunya, dengue, Japanese encephalitis, lymphatic filariasis and zika virus. Mosquito borne diseases are a leading killer of people and animals in developing countries. The resurgence of diseases and the economic impact caused has brought mosquito control to the forefront. There are 3 mosquitos' genera which are vectors of these diseases, viz. Anopheles, Aedes and Culex, among these the day biting mosquito *Ae. aegypti* and *Ae. albopictus* has become important vectors to two important disease namely Dengue and Zika virus. These diseases have alone been responsible for bringing about morbidity in the large population around the world. *Cx. quinquefasciatus* is a vector of Chikungunya, which is a viral affection. It's widely spared distribution across various countries. Malaria caused by *An. stephensi* and *An. arabiensis* still affects large population in developing world. For control of emerging and reemerging mosquito borne diseases, a sound integrated approach towards comprehensive control is the need of hour which could produce sustained effect. The reemergence of mosquito borne diseases like Zika, DHF and CHIKV coupled with the problem of insecticide resistance has both posed a danger as well as a challenge towards mosquito control. In future novel technologies especially Wolbachia based mosquito control, pesticide nanoemulsions, identification of novel bioactive molecules, and novel bacterial pathogens are the key to success of vector control.

Keywords: Mosquito vector, Zika, Wolbachia, Chikungunya, Biological control

1. Introduction

Vector-borne diseases are medically and economically important to the well being of humans and domesticated animals. In the past these diseases were considered to affect the humans living in tropical environment, but today with these diseases have a cosmopolitan distribution virtually encompassing the entire continent including temperate countries [1]. Vector borne diseases have a major impact on the economic well being of human population. A recent WHO report estimates the economic loss due to vector borne diseases worldwide is to the tune of more than 2.5 billion people in over 100 countries are at risk of contracting dengue alone [30].

There are several parasites transmitted by mosquitoes and other insects. The most common transmitters being mosquitoes, which are vectors of several diseases like malaria, zika, dengue, filariasis, chikungunya, Japanese encephalitis, and yellow fever. Three mosquito genera, viz. Anopheles, Aedes and Culex are primarily the vectors which transmit these diseases. Among these diseases Chikungunya is an arthropod-borne virus transmitted mainly by *Aedes* species mosquitoes. Only the female are infective since they need blood meals for egg formation. Chikungunya virus (CHIKV) is an alphavirus from the *Togaviridae* family, which is transmitted by Aedes mosquitoes, and causes epidemic tropical and subtropical countries [28].

CHIKV is a positive-sense, single-stranded RNA virus of about 11.8 kb. There are three main genotypes, West African, Central/East African (C/EA), and Asian, the names reflecting the initial geo-graphic restriction of each type. Since CHIKV was first isolated in Tanzania in 1952 [23], the disease was mainly confined to localized outbreaks in Asia and Africa, sometimes with hundreds of thousands of cases [6]. In 2005, a C/EA strain of CHIKV, which likely originated in coastal Kenya, spread to islands of the Indian Ocean and India [19]. Since then, CHIKV spread worldwide to cause large out breaks in Southeast and East Asia, as well as many imported cases in travelers returning to non-endemic regions in Europe and North America. This global epidemic affecting millions was unprecedented in its scale and was likely driven by several factors. These include the increased volume of travellers, the widening geographic distribution of the mosquito vectors and the adaptation of the epidemic strain to *Aedes albopictus* [26]. The susceptibility of mosquitoes in non-endemic regions such as Australia [27] and North America [21], and the occurrence of autochthonous outbreaks in Italy [22] and France [10], have shown that CHIKV can no longer be considered as a problem of tropical countries. A recent work has also pointed that CHIKV may be present in severe forms, particularly neurological, which may be fatal [15]. It is also increasingly recognized that there is a significant burden of long-term morbidity due to chronic arthralgia [25]. Chikungunya is currently considered as a real threat in these European and American countries, which are colonized by *Aedes* species mosquitoes [2].

There has been little progress in finding cure for the disease. Chikungunya fever is currently symptomatically treated with antipyretics and non-steroidal anti-inflammatory drugs. There will be a continued search for new antiviral candidates with a clearly defined mechanism of viral inhibition in cell-based systems and significant activity in animal models. Considering the global threat this disease poses the immediate disease control measures solely lies in controlling mosquito population.

Dick, Kitchen and Haddow (1952) reported the first isolations of Zika virus from the blood of a sentinel rhesus monkey and from a pool of *Aedes africanus* mosquitoes in Zika forest, Uganda. Virus surveillance elsewhere has yielded more Zika virus isolations from other species of mosquitoes (Lee, 1969). Zika virus (ZIKV), a little known arbovirus, has gained prominence when it caused a large scale epidemic in the Pacific Island in 2007 [9]. It is a member of the genus *Flavivirus* of the Family Flaviviridae. The virus is a positive single stranded RNA virus with a 10,794 nucleotide genome that is closely related to the Spondweni virus [7]. It was first

http://dx.doi.org/10.5772/63134

isolated from a febrile sentinel monkey in Uganda in 1947, but human ZIKV infection was first reported in 1964. The virus causes dengue-like syndromes such as rash, fever, arthralgia, headache and periorbital pain [24].

Zika is a tropical disease transmitted by day biting mosquito *Aedes aegypti* and like CHIKV was a largely neglected disease, until its high epidemic potential was demonstrated in pacific island of YAP in 2007 [9]. Currently this virus has made its presence in Central and South American countries in 2015 and in Feburary 2016 WHO declared Zika infections as public health emergency [32]. Like many vector-borne diseases, the absence of vaccines and specific treatment against ZIKV means prevention and control relies heavily on vector control measure which is needed in order to develop and implement sound mosquito control program.

2. Integrated vector control

Vector control remains the primary defense against diseases like malaria, dengue fever, Chikungunya, zika viral infections etc. The success of vector control relies on the assumption that vector density is related to disease transmission. Vector control and disease prevention strategies are essentially divided into larval and adult mosquito control

1. Removal of stagnant water/ Treatment with biocide oils to prevent egg

   The best method of mosquito is preventing the development of the eggs into adult mosquitoes, by reducing the source of breeding.

2. Insectides-Treated Bed Nets (ITNs)

   The insecticides that are used for treating bed nets kill mosquitoes, as well as other insects. Only pyrethriods insecticides are approved for use on ITNs, these insecticides have been shown to pose very low health risk to humans and other mammals.

3. Personal production creams/sprays

   These type insecticides used as repellent for some human personal production creams for control of mosquitoes against biting.

4. Biological control

   Potential biological control agents such as fungi, *Bacillus thuringiensis*, nematodes, parasites and kill larval mosquitoes, but they are not efficient for mosquito control and are not widely used, likewise mosquito fish have largely been in effective except few studies.

Mosquito control strategies for *Aedes aegypti*, requires special attention as it has ability to breed in polluted water in addition to fresh water. Further this mosquito bites during day as well as night. *Ae. aegypti* and *Ae. albopictus* also called as tiger mosquitoes are highly dangerous in their spectral capacity of spreading dengue fever, DHF, zika and to a certain extent chikungunya diseases among people across the world. These mosquitoes have adapted themselves to be closely associated with human habitation. These mosquitoes breed in polluted as well as freshwater. They can bite at day as well as night. Their breeding sites, including overhead tanks, water in ditches, unused tyres, container harboring water, and polluted sewage water.

The control of Aedes mosquitoes can be done by removing/cleaning waste water, emptying unused water, keeping neighbor's wood are free of open source water bodies and treatment of open water bodies with chemical/biolarvicides, various personal protection steps can be undertaken like use of skin ointment/repellent, covering your bodies with cloth during day time, use of ITNs bed nets during sleeping, households, mosquito coils and other smoke repellents can reduce biting efficacy, similarly windows, household treatment etc., reduce infection

In several countries public awareness programme are conducted by different government agencies involved in mosquito control. In addition, children in schools can be educated about the ways of controlling breeding of mosquito. These community based programme can be successful in large scale eradiation of mosquito breeding sites.

Natural biological control of mosquitoes essentially targets the larval stages. Several predatory insects nymphs like of dragonflies are like Toxorhynchites each larvae and pupa. In addition like *G. affinis, G. holbrooki, Guppy,* and molly, found in normal/natural stress fishes, lakes are efficient in mosquito control. These are known to be very important organisms in paddy ecosystem and other water intensive crops. In addition other non-specific predators like tadpoles and other aquatic predations can help in biological control of mosquitoes.

Chemical pesticides are used by state and local government agencies to control of public health nuisance/pests dangerous to human health. Chemical pesticides are used as a last resort, to do source reduction of mosquitoes populations or when biological control flexible biological control is not feasible, may require larvicidal treatment to prevent the emergence of adult mosquitoes [20]. Use of larvicides is less controversial than use of adulticides, although use of larvicides may lead to public concern about their effects on untargeted beneficial aquatic arthropods and vertebrates.

Effective adult mosquito control with insecticides requires small droplets that drift through areas where mosquitoes are flying. The droplets that impinge on mosquitoes provide the contact activity necessary to kill them. Adulticide applications, particularly aerial applications and thermal fogging, are quite visible and contribute to public apprehension. Ground Ultra Low Volume (ULV) application may be less alarming than aerial application but is not effective over large or inaccessible areas. This technology is being developed and needs validation under different conditions with different mosquito species before it can be universally used.

Several chemical insecticides have been used in mosquito control, primary they fall into 3 broad categories viz. carbamates, organophosphate and synthetic pyrethriods, those chemical insecticides are the most powerful tool available for control of mosquito. They are highly effective for vector control and a reliable alternative for emergency action when insect pest populations exceed the economic threshold [17]. Despite the hazards of conventional insecticides, some use is unavoidable. However, careful chemical choice and application can reduce ecological damage. An array of chemicals has been developed for the killing purpose of insects. These enter the insect body either by penetrating the cuticles or dermal entry, by inhalation into the tracheal system, or by oral ingestion into the digestive system.

Chemical insecticide may be synthetic or natural products. Natural plant derived products, usually called botanical insecticides, include: alkaloids, including nicotine from tobacco, rotenone and other rotenoids from roots of legumes, pyrethroids from flowers of *Tanacetum cinerariifolium*, neem extracts from *Azadirachta indica.* The other major classes of insecticide are synthetic carbamates (carbaryl, aldicarb, methiocarb, methomyl etc), organophosphates (e.g. chlorpyrifos, dichlorvos, malathion, dimethoate and phorate) and organochlorine (aldrin, DDT, dieldrin and endosulfan etc.). Organochlorine are stable chemicals and persistent in the environment, have a low solubility in water and moderate solubility in organic solvents and accumulate in mammalian fat body. The use of this chemical is banned in many countries and they are unsuitable for use in Integrated Pest Management (IPM). Organophosphate are being less environmentally damaging and non-persistent, are suitable for IPM [11]. Most synthetic insecticides are broad spectrum in action and act on insect nervous system. Owing to its high insecticidal activity, low mammalian toxicity and high photostability pyrethroid insecticides are considered as most successful chemical classes of insecticide [4].

Today, world economy is integrated, which has led to transnational flow of goods, people, knowledge, as well as flow of pests, pathogens and vectors across geographical range where natural control is not available. Such kind of emerging infection diseases have become resurgent like zika viral infection in South America and North America, Ebola in Africa and Dengue, in India. What we thought as diseases we controlled are given becoming a threat to people across the world today.

3. *Wolbachia* in the vector control

A new approach to dengue control has recently been proposed that targets mosquito longevity rather than abundance, through the introduction of a life-shortening strain of the bacterium *Wolbachia pipientis* into *Ae. aegypti* populations [5]. α- proteobacteria is best endosymbiotic bacteria species present in insects and nematodes [13]. They infect diverse several arthropods, this is known to affect reproduction and produce nutrients, provide production against pathogens [12, 14]. Wolbachia is an intracellular inherited bacterium, predicted to naturally infect more than 60% of all insect species worldwide [13] that is able to invade host populations through either the induction of a number of reproductive parasitism traits [18] or by positively influencing host fitness [3].

Wolbachia is cytoplasmically inherited, so, infected females usually give rise to females. CI occurs when infected male mates with normal female. In reserve case the offspring are female multiple wolbachia stains may be present in one insect.

Wolbachia is known reproduce parasite when produces cytoplasmic incompatibility, sex ratio distorters, parthenogenesis [29]. They can also enhance reproduce fitness [8]. Mosquito control CI incompatible mates, in *Ae. aegypti* which in naturally uninfected with wolbachia. Wolbachia infected cell lines developed by embryonic microinjection [16], cathartic produces based vector control strategy have been tested in several regions of the world. The release of Wolbachia infected males is an approach that may suppress/reduce natural mosquito population.

4. Future perspective

Vector control strategy essentially needs to encompass 4 broad strategies 1. Spreading and effective way to contain diseases outbreak. 2. Adult mosquito repellant 3. Larval control in aquatic systems 4. Personal protection gear and tools.

Environmental management is a community based approach to eradicate mosquito breeding sites in their locality. To a large extent this exercise can reduce the mosquito population and is rather an effective strategy in urban and sub-urban areas. This approach has its limitations in villages due to the presence of large open water bodies for irrigation and irrigation systems, also environment such as paddy agroecosystem is a rich reservoir of water and is an ideal breeding ground for mosquitoes natural control by entomophagous predators and predatory fishes contain mosquito population to a large extent.

Adult mosquito management using mosquito repellants, in the form of mosquito coils, mats and liquid vaporizers are still in existence; however these are not a permanent solution to adult mosquitoes as they quickly develop resistance to these insecticides in few years. Use of entomopathogenic nematodes, fungus for adult control has limited success. However a new method/ approach of recombinant genetic transformation of Wolbachia in *Aedes* and *Anopheles* genera has been shown to be a promising method for disrupting mosquito –viral interaction thus can be a substantially reduce the disease progression. Personal protection creams like DEET, and other herbal products are still the better choice for person safety, ITNs have been very successful in the control of *Culex* and *Anopheles* borne diseases, however this is rather ineffective against day biting behavior of *Aedes* genera. Sterile male insect technique has met with only limited success and transgenic mosquitoes carrying dominant lethal genes is another method which is still in its infancy. Research needs to address the dynamics of inheritance of these lethal genes and it should also address the sexual selection of transgenic mosquitos' males to others in order to fully analyse its potential in mosquito control. The recent reemergence of mosquito borne diseases like Zika, DHF and CHIKV coupled with the problem of insecticide resistance has both posed a danger as well as a challenge towards mosquito control. In future novel technologies especially Wolbachia based mosquito control, nano emulsions, identification of novel bioactive molecules, and novel bacterial pathogens are the key to success of vector control.

Author details

Sengodan Karthi and Muthugounder Subramaniam Shivakumar*

*Address all correspondence to: skentomol@gmail.com

Molecular Entomology Laboratory, School of Biosciences, Department of Biotechnology, Periyar University, Salem, Tamil Nadu, India

References

[1] Beugnet F, Marie JL. 2009. Emerging arthropod borne diseases of companion animals in Europe. Veterinary Parasitology, 163:298–305.

[2] Boutin JP, Simon F, Oliver M, Grandadam M, Queyriaux B, Tolou H. 2007. [Marseilles, the Indian Ocean and Chikungunya virus]. Bull Acad Natl Med, 191:785–7.

[3] Brownlie, J.C., Cass, B.N., Riegler, M., Witsenburg, J.J., Iturbe-Ormaetxe, I., McGraw, E.A., and O'Neill, S.L. 2009. Evidence for metabolic provisioning by a common invertebrate endosymbiont, Wolbachia pipientis, during periods of nutritional stress. PLoS Pathog. 5, e1000368.

[4] Casida, J.E., Quistad, G.B., 1995. Pyrethrum Flowers – Production, Chemistry, Toxicology and Uses. Brittonia. 48, 613-614.

[5] Cook, P.E., McMeniman, C.J., and O'Neill, S.L. 2008. Modifying insect population age structure to control vector-borne disease. In Transgenesis and the management of vector-borne disease, S. Aksoy, ed. (Austin, TX: Landes Biosciences)

[6] De Ranitz CM, Myers RM, Varkey MJ, Isaac ZH, Carey DE. 1965. Clinical impressions of chikungunya in Vellore gained from study of adult patients. Indian J Med Res, 53:756–63.

[7] Dick GW, Kitchen SF, Haddow AJ (1952) Zika virus. I. Isolations and serological specificity. Trans R Soc Trop Med Hyg 46: 509–520. doi: 10.1016/0035-9203(52)90042-4

[8] Dobson, S, L.,Rattanadeckul, W., Marsland, E,J.(2004). Fitness advantage and cytoplasmic incompatibility in wolbachia single and superinfected *Aedes albopictus*. Heredity, 93,135-142

[9] Duffy MR, Chen TH, Hancock WT, Powers AM, Kool JL, et al. (2009) Zika virus outbreak on Yap Island, Federated States of Micronesia. N Engl J Med 360: 2536–2543. doi: 10.1056/nejmoa0805715

[10] Grandadam M, Caro V, Plumet S, Thiberge JM, Souares Y, Failloux AB, 2011. Chikungunya virus, southeastern France. Emerg Infect Dis,; 17:910–3.

[11] Gullan, P.J., Cranston, P.S., 2010. The insects: An outline of entomology. Fourth Edition, Blackwell Publishing, Oxford, England.

[12] Hedges, L.M. Brownile, J.C., O'Neill, S.L., Johnson, K.N. (2008). Wolbachia and virus production in insects. Science,322, 702

[13] Hilgenboecker, K., Hammerstein, P., Schlattmann, P., Telschow, A., and Werren, J.H. 2008. How many species are infected with Wolbachia?—A statistical analysis of current data. FEMS Microbiol. Lett. 281, 215–220

[14] Hosokawa, T., Koga, R., Kikuchi, Y., Meng, X-Y., Fukatsu, T. (2010). Wolbachia as a bacteriocyte- associated nutritional mutualist. Proc. Natl.Acad. Sci. USA, 107, 769-774.

[15] Lemant J, Boisson V, Winer A, Thibault L, Andre H, Tixier F, 2008. Serious acute chikungunya virus infection requiring intensive care during the Reunion Island outbreak in 2005–2006. Crit Care Med, 36:2536–41.

[16] Mc Meninman, C.J., Lane, A.M., Cass, B.N., Fong, A.W.C., Sindhu, M., Wang, Y.F., O'Neill, S.L. (2009). Stable introduction of a life shorting Wolbachia: infection into the *Aedes aegypti*. Science, 223,141-143.

[17] Metcalf, R.L., Luckmann, W.H., 1994. Introduction to Insect Pest Management. New York: John Wiley and Sons, Inc. pp. 266.

[18] O'Neill, S.L., Hoffmann, A.A., and Werren, J.H. 1997. Influential passengers: inherited microorganisms and arthropod reproduction (Oxford University Press)

[19] Njenga, MK, Nderitu, L, Ledermann, J. P, Ndirangu, A, Logue, CH, Kelly, CHL, Sang, R, Sergon, K, Breiman, R, Powers, AM. (2008). Tracking epidemic Chikungunya virus into the Indian Ocean from East Africa J. Gen. Virol. 89 (11): 2754–2760.

[20] Rawlings JA, Hendricks KA, Burgess CR, Campman RM, Clark GG, Tabony LJ, Patterson MA. 1998. Dengue surveillance in Texas, Am J Trop Med Hyg,; 59:95-9.

[21] Reiskind MH, Pesko K, Westbrook CJ, Mores CN. 2008. Susceptibility of Florida mosquitoes to infection with chikungunya virus. Am J Trop Med Hyg, 78:422–5.

[22] Rezza G, Nicoletti L, Angelini R, Romi R, Finarelli AC, Panning M, 2007. Infection with chikungunya virus in Italy: an outbreak in a temperate region. Lancet,370:1840–6.

[23] Robinson MC. 1955. An epidemic of virus disease in Southern Province, Tanganyika Territory, in 1952–53. I. Clinical features. Trans R Soc Trop Med Hyg, 49:28–32.

[24] Simpson DI (1964) Zika Virus Infection in Man. Trans R Soc Trop Med Hyg 58: 335–338.

[25] Sissoko D, Malvy D, Ezzedine K, Renault P, Moscetti F, Ledrans M, 2009. Post-epidemic Chikungunya disease on Reunion Island: course of rheumatic manifestations and associated factors over a 15-month period. PLoS Negl Trop Dis, 3:389.

[26] Tsetsarkin KA, Vanlandingham DL, McGee CE, Higgs S. 2007. A single mutation in chikungunya virus affects vector specificity and epidemic potential. PLoS Pathog, 3: 201.

[27] Van den Hurk AF, Hall-Mendelin S, Pyke AT, Smith GA, Mackenzie JS. 2010. Vector competence of Australian mosquitoes for chikungunya virus. Vector Borne Zoonotic Dis, 10:489–95.

[28] Weaver SC, Osorio JE, Livengood JA, Chen R, Stinchcomb DT. 2005. Chikungunya virus and prospects for a vaccine. Expert Rev Vaccines, 11:1087–101.

[29] Werren,J.H., Baldo, L.,& Clark, M. E. (2008).Wolbachia; master manipulation of invertebrate biology. Nat. Rev. Microbial., 6, 741-751.

[30] WHO (2014). Vector Borne Diseases. http://www.who.int/campaigns/world-health-day/2014/vector-borne-diseases/en/

[31] WHO (2012). Global Strategy for Dengue Prevention and Control: 2012–2020http://www.who.int/denguecontrol/control_strategies/en/

[32] WHO (2016). http://www.who.int/entity/mediacentre/news/statements/2016/2nd-emergency-committee-zika/en/index.html

Chapter 8

Utilization of Fruit Peel Wastes for the Management of Chikungunya Vector, *Aedes aegypti*

Sarita Kumar, Monika Mishra, Aarti Sharma and Radhika Warikoo

Additional information is available at the end of the chapter

http://dx.doi.org/10.5772/64430

Abstract

Chikungunya, a widely spread viral disease transmitted to human beings by *Aedes aegypti*, is on rise in India, Africa and Asian subcontinent since last decade. Although chemical insecticides are used at a large scale for the control of Chikungunya vector, their applications have led to several undesirable effects including insecticide resistance, revival of pests species, appearance of secondary pests, environmental pollution, noxious hazards to human beings and non-target organisms forcing investigators to explore unconventional alternate strategies. As an environment-friendly approach, there is increased attention to devise and adopt suitable methods to utilize wastes as value-added products to reduce the problem of environmental pollution. Consequently, the larvicidal and adult irritant potential of hexane and petroleum ether peel extracts of three different *Citrus* species, *C. limetta*, *C. sinensis* and *C. Limon*, were assessed against *Ae. aegypti*. The results showed the larvicidal potential of all the three peels, *C. limetta* peel extracts exhibiting the least activity. Furthermore, hexane extracts were more effective than petroleum ether extracts, *C. sinensis* peels hexane extract being most effectual ($LC_{50,}$ 39.51 ppm) while petroleum ether peels extract of *C. limon* was the most effective larvicide with LC_{50} value of 51.25 ppm. All the extracts also exhibited significant elicit response and irritant potential against adults signifying their potential role in reduced mosquito bites and disease transmission. The qualitative phytochemical analysis of the extracts showed presence of certain components suggesting their probable role in bioefficacy of extracts. Further studies are needed to isolate and identify the active ingredient to formulate strategies for mosquito control.

Keywords: *Aedes aegypti*, citrus, larvicidal, peel waste, repellent

1. Introduction

Mosquitoes and the related mosquito-borne diseases are a growing menace around the globe. Prevalence of mosquito-borne diseases is one of the world's most health hazardous problems.

Several mosquito species belonging to genera *Culex, Anopheles* and *Aedes* are vectors for the pathogens of various diseases like filariasis, Japanese encephalitis, malaria, dengue, dengue haemorrhagic fever, yellow fever and Chikungunya [1]. *Ae. aegypti,* the primary carrier for viruses, that cause dengue and Chikungunya fever, is prevalent over wide regions of the tropical and subtropical world. Currently, no effectual vaccine is offered for dengue and Chikunguya fever. Recently, Zika virus disease transmitted by *Aedes* mosquitoes, especially *Ae. aegypti* in tropical world, has been the cause of concern in the world. In today's scenario, the only approach that can be employed to reduce the incidence of *Aedes*-borne diseases is by vector control, which is recurrently reliant on the application of conventional synthetic chemical insecticides [2].

Ae. aegypti, thus has engrossed extensive interest at universal level because of rapid spread of these diseases. Chikungunya is primarily centred across the urban and peri-urban areas, having severe effects in the Asian subcontinent. WHO reports state the massive-fold increase in the number of reported cases over the last decade. Also, the unavailability of a vaccine against the disease further makes the scenario graver.

The first documented outbreak of Chikungunya took place in 1952 in Southern Tanzania, East Africa [3]. Subsequently, epidemics were recorded soon in several other countries : Cambodia, Thailand, Philippines, India, Vietnam, Burma and Sri Lanka. Ever since 2003, there have been outbreaks in the islands of the Pacific Ocean, including Comoros, Mauritius, Madagascar and Reunion Island [4].

The increasing population of Chikungunya vector has urged scientists to come up with effective methods of mosquito control. Several methods have been adopted for controlling mosquito population. In the past, control measures for insect pests and disease vectors utilizing synthetic organic chemical insecticides have caused development of resistance to these insecticides in the disease vector of Chikungunya and dengue fever [5]. It has been reported that insecticide resistance may develop due to changes in the biochemical machinery of mosquitoes, resulting in the quick detoxification or appropriation of the insecticide, or because of the mutation in the target site inhibiting its interaction with insecticide [6]. Progressively, the problem of insecticide resistance is augmenting leading to collapse of many vector control programs. Moreover, the recurrent use of insecticides to manage insect pests and vectors is causing deterioration of the ecosystem [7]. These insecticides are thus, now not a preferred choice for mosquito control because of the environmental degradation they usher. Thus, scientists are now on the look-out for alternative strategies to circumvent the problems posed by the use of synthetic chemical-based insecticides.

Botanicals are one such alternative; researchers are banking upon to alleviate these problems. Although using botanicals seems to be a relatively newer form of mosquito control but its history dates back to the first century AD when a Greek philosopher, Pliny the Elder, wrote "Natural History" and recorded all the pest control methods known at that time. Simultaneously, the Chinese discovered the use of *Chrysanthemum* flowers as an effective insecticide and many others reported a few important phytochemical insecticides, including pyrethrum, derris, quassia, nicotine, hellebore, anabasine, azadirachtin, d-limonene, camphor and turpentine, widely used earlier in developed countries before the introduction of synthetic organic insecticides.

Though with the advent of DDT in 1939, the researchers' quest for mosquito control agents was over and phytochemicals saw their downfall, yet there was a re-focus on phytochemicals because of several problems faced due to injudicious and over application of synthetic insecticides in nature. The scientists have always appreciated the easily biodegradable nature of the phytochemicals leading to no ill-effects on non-target organism. Almost two decades back, phytochemicals could make up only 1 % of world's pesticide market but now, there is a continuous rise in the use of these environment-friendly chemicals.

By definition, phytochemicals are non-nutritive plant chemicals with defensive characteristics. They assist the plants to endure the incessant selection pressure from herbivorous pests, predators and other environmental factors. They are known to be the chemical factories of nature, producing many chemicals, some of which have medicinal and pesticidal properties [8]. Researchers have identified several groups of phytochemicals which possess insecticidal activities. It has been reported that approximately 2000 plant species produce secondary metabolites of importance in pest control programs [9]. Amongst these plant species, metabolites of approximately 344 species have been reported to have a range of activity against mosquitoes [10]. In 2000, Liu et al. suggested these natural plant products as possible alternatives to synthetic chemical insecticides [11]. Some of such phytochemicals include alkaloids, steroids, terpenoids, essential oils and phenolic compounds. The intensity of the insecticidal effect of a particular plant is not static and varies with plant species, mosquito species, geographical varieties, part of the plant used, extraction method adopted, etc. Bio-pesticides provide an alternative to synthetic pesticides as they are effective, easily available, safe for manufacturers and users, biodegradable, inexpensive and environment-friendly.

Recently, there is always an increased attention in bringing useful products from waste materials and fruit wastes are no exceptions. With the increase in production of processed fruit products, the amount of fruit wastes generated is increasing enormously. Citrus is one of the most important commercial fruit crops grown in all continents of the world, the fruits primarily used by juice processing industries while the peels are considered a waste material [12]. Since the juice yield of citrus is less half of the fruit weight, enormous quantity of peel wastes are formed every year. Unfortunately, the peels though perishable and seasonal, they pose a big problem of disposal to the processing industries and pollution monitoring agencies. There is a growing interest to adopt appropriate methods for utilizing them for the conversion into value-added products and improve the overall economics of processing units and reduce the problem of environmental pollution considerably.

Recycling of fruit waste is one of the most imperative means of exploiting it in a number of pioneering and ground-breaking ways leading to the yield of novel products and meeting the requirements of indispensable products required in pharmaceutical industry. The reports are available which confirmed the presence of nutrients and several secondary metabolites in the citrus peels in high magnitude. This clearly indicates the probable use of citrus peel products as drugs and harmless alternate to synthetic chemicals. Consequently, citrus plants have attracted the attention of many workers, and thus organic extracts or essential oils of the leaves and fruit peels are under investigations for various purposes, especially against control of mosquitoes. Suitable methods have to be adopted to utilize them for the conversion into value-added products to improve the overall economics of processing units and reduce the problem of environmental pollution considerably [13]. Many plants have been found to contain chemicals, which are helpful for the control of insects and are useful for field applications in mosquito control programs [14]. Limonene isolated from abraded fresh peels of *Citrus aurantium* has been investigated for its toxicity against larvae of *Cx. quinquefasciatus* and found effective [15]. In 2006, Lee assessed the larvicidal efficacy of *Citrus bergamia* essential oil against *Ae. aegypti* and *Cx. Pipiens* [16], while Amer and Mehlhorn investigated essential oil extracted from *C. limon* against three mosquito species : *Ae. aegypti, Cx. quinquefasciatus* and *Anopheles stephensi* [17].

It is well known that the approach to combat mosquito-borne diseases largely relies on interruption of the disease transmission cycle by either targeting the mosquito larvae at breeding sites through spraying of stagnant water or by killing/repelling the adult mosquitoes using insecticides. Thus, investigations were carried out to explore the efficient anti-mosquito potential of citrus peels obtained from three species of *Citrus* : *C. limetta, C. limon* and *C. sinensis* to control *Ae. aegypti* at larval stage and to repel at adult stage keeping in mind that such a study would not only devise alternate strategies for mosquito control but also would focus towards recycling of wastes, managing littering and waste-related environmental degradation.

2. Review of literature

Citrus plants have attracted the attention of many scientists. Consequently, researchers have carried out investigations on the organic extracts and essential oils extracted from the leaves and fruit peels of citrus plants against different species of insect pests including mosquitoes [18–21]. There are reports available which confirm the larvicidal and repellent activities of the essential oil isolated from *C. sinensis* against *Ae. aegypti* mosquitoes [22].

The larvicidal efficacy of *C. sinensis* peels has been documented against various species of mosquitoes [21]. They reported the respective LC_{50} and LC_{90} values of 58.25 and 298.31 ppm when the larvae of *An. subpictus* were exposed to the chloroform extract of *C. sinensis* peels. On the other hand, assays with methanol extract of *C. sinensis* peels resulted in lower LC_{50} and LC_{90} values of 38.15 and 184.67 ppm, respectively against the larvae of *Cx. tritaeniorhynchus*. The effectiveness of the ethanolic extracts of the *C. sinensis* has been established by Amusan et al. against the larvae of *Ae. aegypti* [23]. Likewise, Michaelakis et al. reported the strong toxicity of essential oils extracted from peels of *C. limon* and *C. sinensis* against larvae of *Cx. pipiens* resulting in the LC_{50} values ranging from 30.1 to 51.5 mg/l, respectively [24]. Earlier investigations have shown that the peel oil extracts of *C. sinensis, C. aurantium* and *C. limon* possessed outstanding larvicidal potential against *Cx. quinquefasciatus* with lemon peel oil exhibiting the maximum larvicidal efficacy [18,19]. The volatile extracts of *C. sinensis* and *C. aurantifolia* (lime) peels were also observed to have cidal activity against mosquitoes [25].

http://dx.doi.org/10.5772/64430

It has been reported earlier that phytochemicals play a foremost role in the mosquito control programmes. Different secondary metabolites of plants, such as alkaloids, steroids, phenolics, terpenoids, saponins, essential oil, etc., are coupled with an extensive range of biological activities. Marston et al. have reported the efficacy of prenylated xanthones, tetracyclic phenols and saponins in controlling the mosquito *Ae. aegypti* [26]. Likewise, the presence of carbohydrates, saponins, phytosterols, phenols, flavonoids and tannins has been observed in the plant extract exhibiting mosquito larvicidal activity [27]. Furthermore, the citrus fruit peel has been found to be a rich source of flavanones and many polymethoxylated flavones, rare in other plants [28]. Kumar et al. have showed the presence of alkaloids, flavonoids and terpenoids in the petroleum ether extracts of *C. sinensis* peels [29]. Table 1 summarizes the larvicidal activity of certain *Citrus* species against different species of mosquitoes.

S. no.	Plant species	Plant product	Mosquito species	Reference
1.	*Citrus aurantium*	Fruit peel oil	*Cx. quinquefasciatus*	Mwaiko (1992)
2.	*Citrus limon*	Fruit peel oil	*Cx. pipiens*	Dakhil and Morsy (1999) Shalaby et al. (1998)
3.	*Citrus sinensis*	Essential oil	*Cx. pipiens molestus*	Traboulsi et al. (2002)
4.	*Citrus reticulata*	Seed extracts	*Cx. quinquefasciatus; Ae. aegypti*	Sumroiphon et al. (2006)
5.	*Citrus sinensis*	Crude peel extracts	*Cx. tritaeniorhynchus, An. subpictus*	Bagavan et al. (2008)
6.	*Citrus sinensis, Citrus limon, Citrus aurantium*	Enantiomers and essential oils	*Cx. pipiens*	Michaelakis et al. (2009)
7.	*Citrus grandis; Citrus mitis, Citrus jhambiri, Citrus paradise, Citrus pseudolimon*	Seed extract	*Ae. albopictus*	Akram et al. (2010)
8.	*Citrus limetta*	Fruit peel extract	*Ae. aegypti*	Kumar et al. (2011c)
9.	*Citrus sinensis*	Leaf extract	*Ae. aegypti*	Kumar et al. (2012)

Table 1. Larvicidal activity of certain *Citrus* species against different species of mosquitoes

3. Materials and methods

3.1. Collection of the larvae and adults of *Ae. aegypti*

The present investigations employ the Chikungunya fever mosquito, *Ae. aegypti* that originated from fields of Delhi and surrounding areas. The larvae were collected from seven locations spread across Delhi and NCR (National Capital Region) (Figure 1). The locations selected were:

- **Okhla, New Delhi** (latitude: 28° N 34′ 2.583″, longitude: 77° E 17′ 32.039″, altitude: 214 m)
- **Alipur, New Delhi** (latitude : 28° N 48′, longitude : 77° E 8′ 59.999″, altitude : 211 m)
- **Dwarka, New Delhi** (latitude: 28° N 35′ 31.704″, longitude: 77° E 2′ 45.773″, altitude: 212 m)
- **Faridabad, Haryana** (latitude: 28° N 24′ 32.08″, longitude: 77° E 19′ 4.041″, altitude: 205 m)
- **Shahdara, New Delhi** (latitude: 28° N 41′ 10.29″, longitude: 77° E 16′ 29.987″, altitude: 211 m)
- **Noida, Uttar Pradesh** (latitude: 28° N 35′ 12.99″, longitude: 77° E 20′ 27.61″, altitude: 201 m)
- **Ghaziabad, Uttar Pradesh** (latitude: 28° N 38′ 11″, longitude: 77° E 25′ 38.1″, altitude: 384 m)

The larvae and adults collected from different locations were brought to the laboratory. The stages were critically observed and those of *Aedes* were segregated and bought back to the laboratory for rearing.

3.2. Laboratory colonization and maintenance of *Ae. aegypti*

The colony of *Ae. aegypti* was maintained in an insectary under controlled conditions of 28 ± 1°C, 80 ± 5% relative humidity and 14:10 light/ dark photoperiod [30]. Adult mosquitoes were kept in screened cloth cages (45 cm × 40 cm × 40 cm) with a long cloth sleeve on one side to prevent the escape of any mosquito from the cage. A wet cotton pad was kept on the top of each cage to provide water to the mosquitoes. Deseeded, water-soaked split raisins kept in a Petri plate were placed in the cage, primarily as a source of food for the male mosquitoes. Female mosquitoes were provided with blood meal on alternate days by keeping a restrained albino rat in the cage for at least 2 h during the day. The day following blood meal, an ovitrap consisting of an enamel bowl lined on all sides with the Whatman filter paper and half-filled with dechlorinated water was kept in the cage for the collection of eggs. Dechlorinated water was prepared by storing tap water in large plastic buckets for 24 h. The strips of the filter paper laden with the eggs were taken out on every alternate day and kept moist for 2 days to allow embryonation of eggs. A few strips were subsequently dried and stored in sterilized bottles. The bottles were stocked in the refrigerator at 4°C. The eggs, thus stored, were viable for at least 6 months. Whenever required, the stored egg strips were dipped into deoxygenated water, which was prepared by boiling distilled water in an Erlenmeyer flask and then cooling it without access to the air. This resulted in synchronous and immediate hatching of larvae within 20– 25 min.

The remaining egg strips were dipped in the dechlorinated water for maintenance of culture. The newly emerged larvae were transferred in dechlorinated water-filled enamel trays (25 cm × 30 cm × 5 cm) for rearing. Each day, food consisting of finely ground dog biscuits and yeast (3:1 by weight) was provided to the larvae. Paramount care was taken to prevent scum formation on the surface of water. The larval period of *Ae. aegypti* comprising four instars, lasted for 9– 10 days. Pupae formed were isolated into an enamel bowl containing water which was then kept in the cloth cage for adult emergence. Blood meal was provided to the female mosquitoes on the third day after emergence.

http://dx.doi.org/10.5772/64430

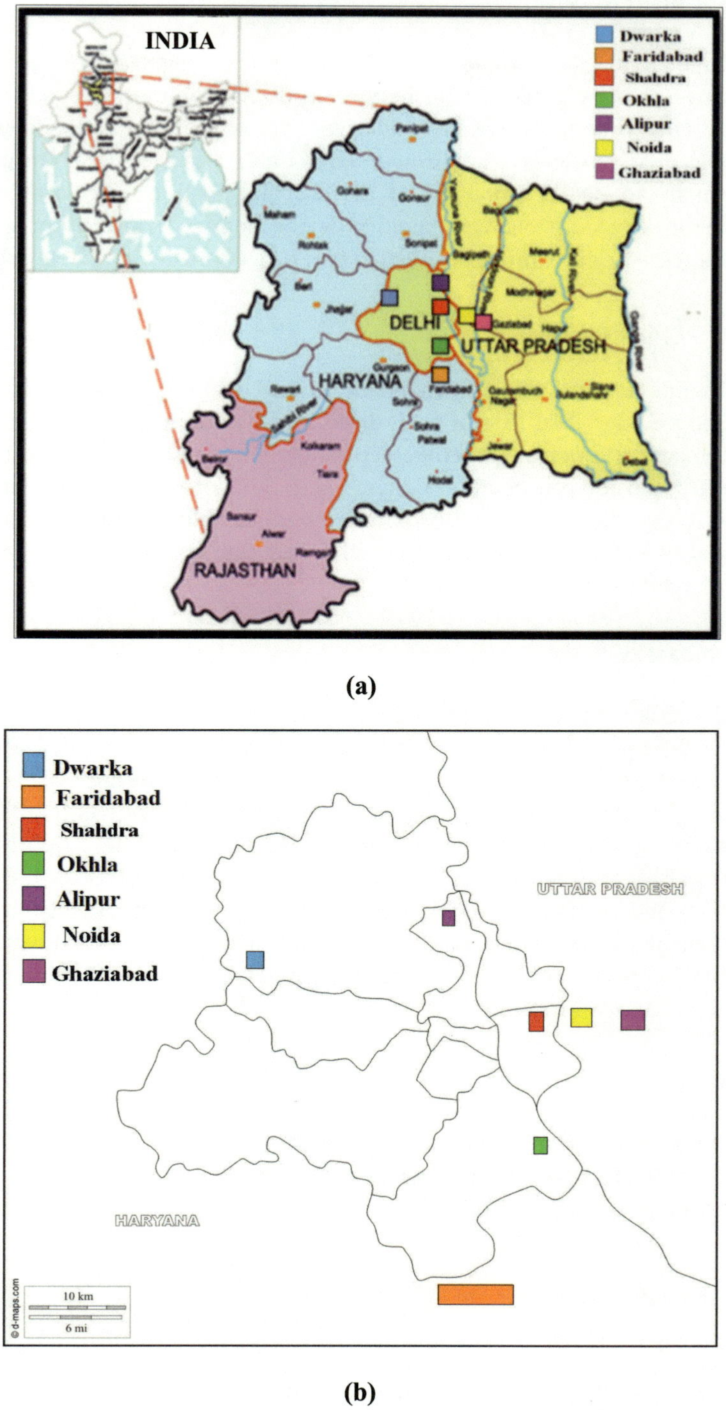

Figure 1. Areas selected in Delhi and NCR for the collection of *Aedes aegypti* larvae:(a) overview; (b) enlarged view.

3.3. Collection of plant material

The fruits of three citrus plants *C. sinensis*, *C. limon* and *C. limetta* were gathered from the surrounding areas of New Delhi, India in the sterilized polythene bags. The peels were separated from all the three species of fruits and were thoroughly washed with tap water. Care was taken to clean dust, particles or any unwanted material stuck to them. The peels were also observed cautiously to detect any kind of disease or infection. The infected peels were discarded while the selected peels were kept for drying under shade at room temperature (27 ± 2°C). The peels were dried completely ensuring to prevent fungal or bacterial growth.

3.4. Preparation of peel extract

The dried peels were mechanically grinded using a small blender. The grounded material was sieved to get fine powder. The 15 g of each dried and powdered citrus peels was extracted with 200 ml of hexane and petroleum ether, separately. The extraction was carried out for 8 h per day and continued for consecutive 3 days, using Soxhlet extractor at a temperature not exceeding the boiling point of the solvent. The six extracts obtained were concentrated using a vacuum evaporator at 45°C under low pressure and stored in a refrigerator at 4°C as the stock solution of 1000 ppm for further use.

3.5. Larvicidal bioassay

The larvicidal bioassay was performed at 28 ± 1°C on the *Ae. aegypti* early fourth instars in agreement with the methodology described by WHO with minor modifications [31]. The graded series of each peel extract was prepared using ethanol as the solvent. The early fourth instars of *Ae. aegypti* were separated, in groups of 20, in plastic bowls filled with 99 ml of distilled water. The larvae were transferred to a glass jar containing 1 ml of the particular concentration of extract added to 100 ml of distilled water. For each dilution, four simultaneous replicates were carried out making a total of 80 larvae for each extract concentration. On the other hand, in controls, ethanol was added to water instead of peel extract. During the exposure period, the larvae were not provided with any food. The dead and moribund larvae were recorded after 24 h as larval mortality.

3.6. Data analysis

The tests with more than 20% mortality in control assays and 20% pupae formed were rejected and performed again. In case, the control mortality ranged between 5% and 20%, it was rectified using Abbott's formula [32].

$$\text{Corrected mortality} = \frac{\%\ \text{Test Mortality} - \%\ \text{Control Mortality}}{100 - \%\ \text{Control Mortality}} \times 100$$

The data was subjected to the regression analysis using computerized SPSS 18.0 Programme. The LC_{50} and LC_{90} values with 95% fiducial limits were calculated in each bioassay to measure difference between the test samples. Other statistical parameters, such as standard error and regression coefficient, were also recorded.

3.7. Contact irritancy assays

Whatman filter paper circles were impregnated with 50 ppm hexane and petroleum ether peel extracts of *C. sinensis, C. limon* and *C. limetta,* separately. These papers were completely dried and used afresh for contact irritancy assays. Each paper was placed on a glass plate and a Perspex funnel with a hole on the top was kept inverted over them. The 3-day- old unfed female adults of *Ae. aegypti* were separated. Single female was released inside the funnel on the paper. The opening on the top of funnel was plugged with a cotton swab. The adult was left undisturbed to settle for 3 min after which the time taken for the first take-off flight was recorded. The assay was continued for 15 min during which the total number of flights undertaken by that mosquito was scored. Similar parallel control tests were performed with ethanol-impregnated papers. Each treatment had three replicates. Data was analysed and the relative irritability of the extract in each case was calculated with respect to control.

3.8. Phytochemical analysis

All the extracts were subjected to preliminary screening of phytochemical investigation and the components in each extract were identified using standard protocols as documented by Harborne et al. [33]. Various qualitative tests were performed to discover the presence of alkaloids, phenolic compounds, carbohydrates, flavonoids, tannins, phlobatannins, saponins and terpenoids in the extracts.

4. Results

Present investigations were performed with an objective to formulate a safe and environment-friendly strategy for minimization of waste in fruit juice processing industry by employing citrus fruit peel waste as the larvicidal agent against *Ae. aegypti*. Keeping this in view, the hexane and petroleum ether extracts of *C. Sinensis, C. limon* and *C. limetta* peels were assessed for their larvicidal and irritant potential against early fourth instar larvae and non-bleed fed females of *Ae. aegypti*. The comparative result of larvicidal bioassays of peel extracts performed on early fourth instar larvae of *Ae. aegypti* with hexane and petroleum ether extracts of *C. sinensis, C. limon* and *C. limetta* peels are presented in Tables 2– 4, respectively. The results prove and establish the efficacy of all the extracts of citrus peels against the mosquito larvae.

Our investigations showed that the hexane extracts of peels were more effective than petroleum ether extracts irrespective of the citrus species. The hexane extract of *C. sinensis* peels proved to be more effectual larvicidal agent against *Ae. aegypti* resulting in LC_{50} values as low as 39.51 ppm. Nevertheless, petroleum ether peels extract of *C. limon* was the most effective larvicidal agent against *Ae. aegypti* with LC_{50} value of 51.25 ppm, while that of *C. limetta* peel wastes showed least activity exhibiting LC_{50} value of 145.50 ppm. All treatments resulted in complete mortality without any pupa or adult emergence. The control or untreated groups did not show any mortality within 24 h. The larvae developed into pupae and then adults within 48–72 h (Figure 2).

Extraction solvent	LC_{50} (ppm)	95% Fiducial limits	LC_{90} (ppm)	95% Fiducial limits	S.E.	χ^2 (*df*)	Regression coefficient
Hexane	39.51	35.22–43.66	61.90	54.73–74.99	0.97	2.16 (5)	6.57
Petroleum ether	55.58	50.22–60.62	85.05	75.56–104.51	1.15	7.06 (5)	6.93

Table 2. Larvicidal activity of extracts prepared from the peels of *Citrus sinensis* against early fourth instars of *Aedes aegypti*

Extract	LC_{50} (ppm)	95% Fiducial limits	LC_{90} (ppm)	95% Fiducial limits	S.E.	χ^2 (*df*)	Regression coefficient
Hexane	46.08	40.10–52.07	85.34	72.83–109.29	0.68	4.78 (5)	4.78
Petroleum ether	51.25	45.37–57.83	93.50	79.01–122.97	0.71	3.36 (6)	4.90

Table 3. Larvicidal activity of extracts prepared from the peels of *Citrus limon* against early fourth instars of *Aedes aegypti*

Extraction solvent	LC_{50} (ppm)	95% Fiducial limits	LC_{90} (ppm)	95% Fiducial limits	S.E.	χ^2 (*df*)	Regression coefficient
Hexane	96.15	83.52–112.11	163.27	139.21–241.30	1.08	7.58 (6)	5.57
Petroleum ether	145.50	118.05–180.58	371.48	278.83–596.47	0.47	6.52 (4)	3.14

Table 4. Larvicidal activity of extracts prepared from the peels of *Citrus limetta* against early fourth instars of *Aedes aegypti*

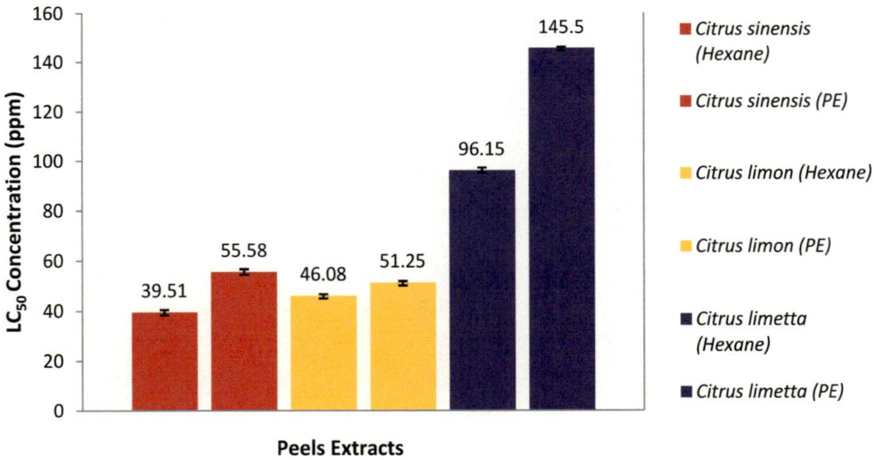

Figure 2. Comparison of LC_{50} value of hexane and petroleum ether extracts prepared from the peels of *Citrus sinensis, Citrus limon* and *Citrus limetta* against early fourth instars of *Aedes aegypti.*

http://dx.doi.org/10.5772/64430

When the females of *Ae. aegypti* were subjected to contact irritancy assays, a significant response was observed (Table 5). The results revealed the more irritant potential of petroleum ether extracts as compared to hexane extracts. The petroleum ether extract of *C. limon* was found to be the most effective against *Ae. aegypti* with first time of flight recorded as 14s with maximum irritability effect of 25-fold (Table 5).

Solvent of extraction	Mean time lapse before first take-off (in s)	Mean no. of take- offs for females (in 15 min)	Relative irritability
	Control		
–	410.00 (258.30)	1.00 (1.00)	1.00
	(a) *Citrus sinensis*		
Hexane	29.66 (33.8)	6.00 (4.35)	6.00
Petroleum ether	38.60 (21.00)	10.00 (2.00)	10.00
	(b) *Citrus limon*		
Hexane	39.33 (35.55)	12.00 (11.26)	12.00
Petroleum ether	14.00 (4.00)	25.33 (9.60)	25.33
	(c) *Citrus limetta*		
Hexane	66.33 (54.81)	18.30 (6.50)	18.30
Petroleum ether	53.00 (13.07)	18.60 (4.16)	18.60

Figures in parentheses indicate standard deviation.

Table 5. Response of of non-blood fed females of *Ae. aegypti* to papers impregnated with extracts of *Citrus sinensis*, *Citrus limon* and *Citrus limetta* in the contact irritancy assays

S. no.	Phytochemical constituents	Hexane extract	Petroleum ether extract
1	Alkaloid	–	+
2	Carbohydrates	–	–
3	Saponins	–	–
4	Phenolic compounds	–	–
5	Tannins	–	–
6	Flavonoids	+	+
7	Terpenoids	+	+
8	Phlobatannins	–	–

Table 6. Phytochemical screening of *Citrus* peels

The preliminary qualitative phytochemical analysis of the peel extracts of all the three *Citrus* sp. discovered the occurrence of terpenoids and flavonoids in both the hexane and petroleum ether extracts (Table 6). Other components, i.e., carbohydrates, phenolic compounds, saponins, tannins and phlobatannins were not noticed in any of these extracts. Nevertheless, the petroleum ether extract exhibited alkaloids, the presence of which was not observed in the hexane extracts.

5. Discussion

It is well documented that the control of mosquito-borne diseases can be achieved either at adult stage preventing mosquitoes to bite human beings by using repellents/irritants or at larval stage causing mortality at a large scale in the breeding areas. Nonetheless, the widespread use of synthetic insecticides has caused environmental risks and the development of insecticide resistance in the vector species. The adverse impact of insecticides has caused concern and necessitated the search and development of environmentally safe, biodegradable, economically effective and indigenous methods for mosquito control, which can be employed with least care by human beings and communities [1].

A number of reports documented in the field of mosquito control reveal the worthiness of diverse phytochemicals procured from various plant species against different mosquito species. Sukumar et al. made an extensive review of botanical derivatives which have been investigated against mosquitoes [10]. They reported a large number of plant extracts which possess cidal or repellent activities against mosquito vectors, but indicated that very few plant products have shown practical value for mosquito control. Plants are known to be rich sources of complex mixtures of bioactive compounds that can be used to develop environmentally safe vector and pest-managing agents. Nevertheless, natural pesticides derived from plants are a promising tool especially for targeting mosquitoes in larval stage [21]. Our experiments reveal the hexane extracts of the peels of all the three *Citrus* species were highly effective against *Ae. aegypti* as compared to petroleum ether extracts.

Very few reports are available regarding larvicidal and contact irritancy of citrus peels against *Ae. aegypti*. Our results are in agreement with that of Murugan et al. who had tested the efficacy of *C. sinensis* ethanolic peel extract against *Ae. aegypti* and *Cx. quinquefasciatus* and found it to be more effective against *Ae. aegypti* having LC_{50} value of 92.27 ppm whereas against *Cx. quinquefasciatus* the value reported was 244.70 ppm [34]. The essential oils extracted from peels of *C. limon* and *C. sinensis* have been reported to exhibit strong toxicity against larvae of *Cx. pipiens* with the LC_{50} values ranging from 30.1 to 51.5 mg/l [24]. Akram et al. had found extracts prepared from the seeds of rough lemon and lemon as effective larvicides with LC_{50} values of 119.993 and 137.258 ppm, respectively, after 24 h of exposure and 108.85 and 119.853 ppm, respectively, after 48 h of exposure [35]. The volatile peel extracts of *C. sinensis* and *C. aurantifolia* (lime) were also reported to have insecticidal activity against mosquitoes [25].

Our studies also showed significant irritant potential of petroleum ether extract of *C. limon* against *Ae. aegypti* as compared to *C. sinensis* and *C. limetta* extracts. Similar repellency behaviour in *Ae. aegypti* was reported by Kumar et al. when adults were exposed to the leaf extracts of *Parthenium hysterophorus* prepared in different solvents [36]. Essential oils from a few verbenaceae plants have also shown repellent activity against *Ae. aegypti*, *An. stephensi* and

Cx. quinquefasciatus [17]. Similarly repellency of aromatic plants and pure components was studied by Abdallah et al. against *Cx. pipiens molestus* [37]. The potential of volatile oils extracted from turmeric, citronella grass and hairy basil as topical repellents have also been reported against *Ae. aegypti, An. dirus* and *Cx. quinquefasciatus* [38]. Thangam also studied repellent activity of acetonic extracts of four seaweeds *Caulerpa peltata, C. racemosa, C. scalpelliformis* and *Diclyota dichotoma* and eleven mangrove plant samples, *Avicennia marina, A. officinalis, Excoecaria agallocha, Lumnitzera racemosa, Rhizophora apiculata, R. lamarckii, R. mucronata, Salicornia brachiata, Sonneratia apetala, Xylocarpus granatum*, against *Ae. aegypti* out of which he found the stilt root of *Rhizophora apiculata* extract to be most effective [39]. Petroleum ether extract of *Vitex negundo* leaves offered bite protection for 8 h (2 mg/cm^2) by different mosquitoes in the field [40]. This suggests that natural pesticides derived from plants are a promising tool for mosquito control programs.

Earlier studies have showed that phytochemicals play a major role in mosquito control programme. The secondary metabolites of plants (such as steroids, alkaloids, terpenoids, saponins, phenolics, essential oil, etc.) are associated with a wide range of biological activities. Marston et al. have reported the efficacy of prenylated xanthones, tetracyclic phenols and saponins in controlling *Ae. aegypti* [26]. Likewise, the presence of carbohydrates, saponins, phytosterols, phenols, flavonoids and tannins have been observed in the plant extract exhibiting mosquito larvicidal activity [27]. Furthermore, the citrus fruit peel has been found to be a rich source of flavanones and many polymethoxylated flavones, rare in other plants [28].

The present study showed the presence of flavonoids and terpenoids as the common constituents in the hexane and petroleum ether extracts of *Citrus* sp. These results are in conformity with that of Kumar et al. who showed the presence of alkaloids, flavonoids and terpenoids in the petroleum ether extracts of *C. sinensis* peels [29]. The presence of flavonoids and cardiac glycosides in methanol extract of *Lantana camara* leaves and flowers, flavonoids in leaf and terpenoids in the flower of ethanol extract has been shown by Sathish and Maneemegalai [41]. Rawani et al. suggested that the presence of bioactive principles such as steroids, alkaloids, terpenes, saponins, etc. may be responsible for the larvicidal properties of crude extracts of three plants, *viz. Carica papaya, Murraya paniculata* and *Cleistanthus collinus* against *Cx. quinquefasciatus* [42]. Vinayachandra et al. concluded that either the presence of saponins, phenolics, steroids or terpenoids in the plant extracts of *Knema attenuata* or a combination of two or more of these metabolites might be the cause for larvicidal efficacy against the Indian strains of *An. stephensi* and *Ae. albopictus* [43]. Although our investigations have revealed the occurrence of only two phytochemical constituents, the larvicidal potential of the extracts might be because of the synergistic effects of other phytochemical constituents present in the extracts, identified or unidentified in the present investigation.

6. Conclusion

Our studies have clearly demonstrated that waste peels of citrus fruits can be utilized as the effective agents of mosquito control. The utilization of wastes as beneficial products would not only assist to reduce waste load by managing intractable waste discharge but would also diminish the pollution load and improve the environmental profile of fruit juice processing industry.

Acknowledgements

The authors are grateful to Dr Savithri Singh, Principal, Acharya Narendra Dev College, for providing the laboratory and culture facilities to conduct the experimental work.

Author details

Sarita Kumar*, Monika Mishra, Aarti Sharma and Radhika Warikoo

*Address all correspondence to: saritakumar@andc.du.ac.in

Department of Zoology, Acharya Narendra Dev College, University of Delhi, Delhi, India

References

[1] Mittal PK, Subbarao SK. Prospects of using herbal products in the control of mosquito vectors, ICMR Bulletin. 2003; 33 (1), 1–10.

[2] Malavige GN, Fernando S, Fernando DJ, Seneviratne SL. Dengue viral infections, Postgraduate Medical Journal. 2004; 80, 588–601.

[3] World Health Organization. Chikungunya. 2015. http://www.who.int/mediacentre/factsheets/fs327/en/ (Accessed on September 30, 2015).

[4] National Vector Borne Diseases Control Program. 2015. http://nvbdcp.gov.in/Chikun-main.html (Accessed on August 27, 2015).

[5] World Health Organization. Vector resistance to insecticides. 15th Report of the WHO Expert Committee on Vector Biology and Control. World Health Organization Technical Report Series, 1992; 818, 1–62.

[6] Hemingway J, Hawkes NJ, McCarroll L, Ranson H. The molecular basis of insecticide resistance in mosquitoes. Insect Biochemistry and Molecular Biology; 2004 ; 34, 653–665.

[7] Kranthi KR, Jadhav D, Wanjari R, Russell D. Pyrethroid resistance and mechanisms of resistance in field strains of *Helicoverpa armigera* (Lepidoptera: Noctuidae). Journal of Economic Entomology. 2001 ; 94, 253–263.

[8] Chansang U, Zahiri NS, Bansiddhi J, Boonruad T, Thongsrirak P, Mingmuang J, Benjapong N, Mulla MS. Mosquito larvicidal activity of aqueous extracts of long pepper (*Piper retrofractum* Vahl.) from Thailand. Journal of Vector Ecology. 2005; 30, 195–200.

[9] Ahmed S, Graivge M, Hylin JW, Mitchell WC, Listinger JA. Some promising plant species for use as pest control agents under traditional farming system. In: Schmutterer H, Ascher KRS, editors; Proceedings of 2nd International Neem Conference, Rauischolzhausen, Germany; GTZ, Eschborn, Germany; 1984, p. 565–580.

[10] Sukumar K, Perich MJ, Boombar LR. Botanical derivatives in mosquito control: a review. Journal of American Mosquito Control Association. 1991 ; 7, 210–237.

[11] Liu SQ, Shi JJ, Cao H, Jia FB, Liu XQ, Shi GL. Survey of pesticidal component in plant. In: Entomology in China in 21st Century. Proceedings of 2000 Conference of Chinese Entomological Society; Science & Technique Press, Beijing, China; 2000, p. 1098–1104.

[12] Manthey A, Grohmann K. Phenols in citrus peel by products: concentrations of hydroxycinnamates and polymethoxylated flavones in citrus peel molasses. Journal of Agriculture and Food Chemistry. 2001 ; 49, 3268–3273.

[13] Nand K. Recent advances in the treatment of liquid and solid wastes of food processing industries for biogas production and pollution abatement. In: Proceedings of IV International Food Convention; 1998.

[14] Sujatha CH, Vasuki V, Mariappan T, Kalyanasundaran M, Das PK. Evaluation of plant extracts for biological activity against mosquitoes. International Pest Control. 1988 ; 30: 398–401.

[15] Kassir JT, Mohsen Z-H, Mehdi N-S. Toxic effects of limonene against *Culex quinquefasciatus* Say larvae and its interference with oviposition. Anz Schädlingskde Pflanzenschutz Umweltschutz. 1989 ; 62, 19–22.

[16] Lee HS. Mosquito larvicidal activity of aromatic medicinal plant oils against *Aedes aegypti* and *Culex pipiens pallens*. Journal of American Mosquito Control Association. 2006 ; 22, 292–295.

[17] Amer A, Mehlhorn H. Larvicidal effects of various essential oils against *Aedes, Anopheles* and *Culex* larvae (Diptera, Culicidae). Parasitology Research. 2006 ; 99, 466–472.

[18] Mwaiko GL. Citrus peel oil extracts as mosquito larvae insecticides. East African Medical Journal. 1992 ; 69, 223–226.

[19] Mwaiko GL, Savaeli ZXN. Lemon peel oil extract as mosquito larvicide. East African Medical Journal. 1994 ; 71, 797–799.

[20] Shalaby AA, Allam KAM, Mostafa AA, Fahmy SME. Insecticidal properties of citrus oils against *Culex pipiens* and *Musca domestica*. Journal of the Egyptian Society of Parasitology. 1998 ; 28, 595–606.

[21] Bagavan A, Kamaraj C, Rahuman AA, Elango G, Zahir AA, Pandiyan G. Evaluation of larvicidal and nymphicidal potential of plant extracts against *Anopheles subpictus* Grassi, *Culex tritaeniorhynchus* Giles and *Aphis gossypii* Glover. Parasitology Research. 2008 ; 104, 1109–1117.

[22] Omobuwajo OR, Gbolade AA, Nia R, Adewoyin FB. 11th Napreca Symposium Abstracts. The 11th Symposium of the Natural Product Research Network for Eastern and Central Africa (NAPRECA); 9–12 August 2005; Madagascar, Antananarivo, p. 72.

[23] Amusan AA, Idowu AB, Arowolo FS. Comparative toxicity of bush tea leaves (*Hyptis suaveolens*) and orange peel (*Citrus sinensis*) oil extracts on the larvae of the yellow fever mosquito *Aedes aegypti*. Tanzania Health Research Bulletin. 2005 ; 7, 174–178.

[24] Michaelakis A, Papachristos D, Kimbaris A, Koliopoulos G, Giatropoulos A, Polissiou MG. Citrus essential oils and four enantiomeric pinenes against *Culex pipiens* (Diptera: Culicidae). Parasitology Research. 2009 ; 105, 769–773.

[25] Ezeonu FC, Chidume GI, Udedi SC. Insecticidal properties of volatile extracts of orange peels. Bioresource Technology. 2001 ; 76, 273–274.

[26] Marston A, Maillard M, Hostettmann K. Search for antifungal, molluscicidal and larvicidal compounds from African medicinal plants. Journal of Ethnopharmacology. 1993 ; 38, 215–223.

[27] Gopieshkhanna V, Kannabiran K. Larvicidal effect of *Hemidesmus indicus, Gymnema sylvestre* and *Eclipta prostrata* against *Culex quinquefasciatus* mosquito larva. African Journal of Biotechnology. 2008 ; 6, 307–311.

[28] Ahmad MM, Salim-ur-Rehman IZ, Anjum FM, Sultan JI. Genetic variability to essential oil composition in four citrus fruit species. Pakistan Journal of Botany. 2006 ; 38, 319–324.

[29] Kumar S, Ray A, Kaur J, Samal R, Wahab N, Warikoo R. Efficacy of the ethanolic leaf extracts of citrus plant, *Citrus sinensis* as larvicidal and irritant agent against dengue vector *Aedes aegypti* L. Asian Pacific Journal of Tropical Biomedicine. 2012 ; 3, 152–155.

[30] Kumar S, Warikoo R, Wahab N. Larvicidal potential of ethanolic extracts of dried fruits of three species of peppercorns against different instars of an Indian strain of dengue fever mosquito, *Aedes aegypti* L. (Diptera: Culicidae). Parasitology Research. 2010 ; 107, 901–907.

[31] World Health Organization, Report WHO World Malaria Report. 2005, WHO/ UNICEF, Geneva.

[32] Abbott WB. A method for computing the effectiveness of an insecticide. Journal of Economic Entomology. 1925 ; 18, 265–267.

[33] Harborne JB, Harborne AJ. Phytochemical Methods: A Guide to Modern Techniques of Plant Analysis. Kluwer Academic Publishers, London, UK; 1998.

[34] Murugan K, Mahesh KP, Kovendan K, Amerasan D, Subrmaniam J, Hwanq JS. Larvicidal, pupicidal, repellent and adulticidal activity of *Citrus sinensis* orange peel extract against *Anopheles stephensi, Aedes aegypti* and *Culex quinquefasciatus* (Diptera: Culicidae). Parasitology Research. 2012 ; 6–7. DOI: 10.1007/s00436-012-3021-8.

[35] Akram W, Khan AAA, Hafeez F, Bilal H, Kim YK, Lee J-J. Potential of citrus seed extracts against dengue Fever mosquito, *Aedes albopictus* (skuse) (Culicidae: Diptera). Pakistan Journal of Botany. 2010 ; 42, 3343–3348.

[36] Kumar S, Singh AP, Nair G, Batra S, Seth A, Wahab N, Warikoo R. Impact of *Parthenium hysterophorus* leaf extracts on the fecundity, fertility and behavioural response of *Aedes aegypti.* Parasitology Research. 2011 ; 108, 853-859.

[37] Abdallah FT, Samih EH, Marie T, Khalil T, Naltalie AN, Abir M. Repellency and toxicity of aromatic plant extracts against the mosquito *Culex pipiens molestus* (Diptera: Culicidae). Pest Management Science. 2005 ; 61(6), 1002–1017.

[38] Apiwat T, Steve DWR, Roderic S, Usavadee T, Yenchit T. Repellency of volatile oils from plants against three mosquito vectors. Journal of Vector Ecology. 2001 ; 26(1), 76–82.

[39] Thangam TS, Kathiresan K. Repellency of marine plant extracts against the mosquito *Aedes aegypti.* Pharmaceutical Biology. 1993 ; 31, 321–323.

[40] Karunamoorthi K, Rmunajam S, Rathinasamy R. Evaluation of leaf extracts of *Vitex negundo* L. (Family, Verbenacea) against larvae of *Culex tritaeniorhynchus* and repellent activities on adult vector mosquitoes. Parasitology Research. 2008 ; 103, 545–550.

[41] Sathish KM, Maneemegalai S. Evaluation of larvicidal effect of *Lantana camara* Linn against mosquito species *Aedes aegypti* and *Culex quinquefasciatus.* Advanced Biology Research. 2008 ; 2, 39–43.

[42] Rawani A, Haldar KM, Ghosh A, Chandra G. Larvicidal activities of three plants against filarial vector *Culex quinquefasciatus* Say (Diptera: Culicidae). Parasitology Research, 2009 ; 105, 1411–1417.

[43] Vinayachandra, Shwetha R, Chandrashekar KR. Larvicidal activities of *Knema attenuata* (Hook. f. & Thomson) Warb. (Myristicaceae) extracts against *Aedes albopictus* Skuse and *Anopheles stephensi* Liston. Parasitology Research. 2011 ; 109, 1671–1676.